Is
Pharmacology
Difficult

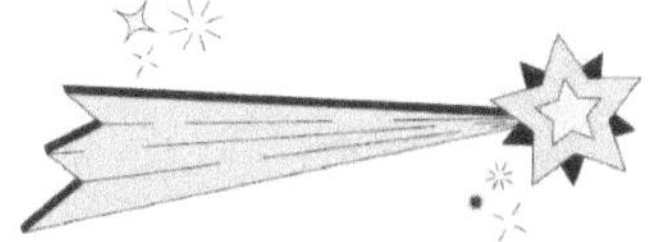

Book 1 (General Pharmacology)
2nd Edition

Radhika Vijay

Mbbs MD Pharmacology
Bikaner, Rajasthan, India

Is

Pharmacology

Difficult

Dedicated to my

beloved late

"Dad"

Foreword

This book marks the joy of the end of "Season 1" of my Podcast, namely

"Is Pharmacology Difficult Podcast". It is a special effort for those

interested in the subject but either not willing to lend an ear or having a

dedicated reading passion or a serious disciplined attitude of a highly

intellectual student (medical, nursing, dental, pharmacy, etc) who stay

away from social media, all sorts of Apps, music internet happenings and

always wrapped up in his/her own cocoon, a true bookworm!

I truly appreciate this behaviour, because I have myself been one of this

kind especially in the days of striving hard for my degrees, and I believe

such an attitude is must to make your dreams come true, so for all those

who love to read and especially want to learn Pharmacology, here you have

this my "Book 1" in the series of "Is Pharmacology Difficult"!

With a slight reflection of the inspiring, informational and witty episodic

linguistic twists and turns and a lot many handmade diagrams, some nice

to learn and read tables, you will be able to comprehend a lot about

General Pharmacology and stay motivated with "Seven steps to success"

quotes by Sir John C. Maxwell all the way through your reading journey!

Don't forget to subscribe to my free

"Pharmacology Further" E-Newsletter

by simply signing up at

https://pharmacologyfurther.substack.com/

Alternatively at:

https://www.ispharmacologydifficult.com .

It contains a lot of updates about drugs, medicines,

Health, from my classroom section

and my podcast updates also.

And now the *Radgin Wiz Writing Desk,*

Simple & Sparkling and Off The Cuff Talks sections

are added to let you all know more!

Table Of Contents

1. Chapter 1.........(Once Upon A Time....To The Present!!)

2. Chapter 2.......(Pharmacokinetics at a Glance-1: Routes of Drug Administration, Dosage Forms, Absorption, Distribution, Biotransformation of drugs)

3. Chapter 3......(Pharmacokinetics at a Glance-2: Elimination Kinetics of Drugs)

4. Chapter 4.......(Pharmacodynamics at a Glance-1: Receptor Theory)

5. Chapter 5......(Pharmacodynamics at a Glance-2: Dose Response Relationship)

6. Chapter 6.........(Pharmacogenetics and Pharmacogenomics)

7. Chapter 7.........(Drug Safety & Toxicology)

Chapter 1

Once Upon A Time....

To The Present!

KEY POINTS:

- *Drug Origin*
- *Evolution of Pharmacology*
- *Discovery of Drugs*
- *Important Definitions*
- *Nature and sources of Drugs and Name of drugs*

Since the past era, humans have always looked forward to and been dependent on plants. Miraculous and magical serendipity lead to the development of most of the plant-derived medicines.

In ancient times, drugs were used raw, with ingredients, amount unknown. The brainy people then once discovered, observed and established the effect of any plant derived material, etc, it was bound to be used repeatedly, irrespective of knowledge of its composition and active moiety.

"EFFECT DOMINATED THE MECHANISM"

Some such wonderful examples include the use of Coffee (Caffeine) by an Arabian convent who was inspired by some weird behaviour of Goats who fed on Coffee Berries. Belladonna (Beautiful lady) extract from mushrooms were used to dilate eye pupils by Professional poisoners. Chinese herb "Ma Huang" was a source of ephedrine to stimulate circulation. Curare was used to paralyse and kill hunted animals for food.Relief of pain was by Morphine (Opium) obtained from Poppy plant juice.Morphine along with similar natural compounds like Cocaine, ethanol were abused due to their addicting potential too!

EVOLUTION OF PHARMACOLOGY

This includes both the old concept of discovery and the modern concept of synthesising drugs.

Drug Discovery is an important process and its study is inevitable.

Drug invention set its feet strong in the field of Synthetic chemistry, i.e. in the Dye industry.

Paul Ehrlich was inspired to establish the presence of chemical receptors in tissues which reacted and "fixed" the dyes. The concept of "Receptors" was harbingered.

 Consistent interest and hard work led to the invention of *Arsphenamine,* later patented as "Salvarsan". Added benefits of the technique were used for treatment of Syphilis.

Gerhard Domagk worked on another dye, "Prontosil" (first chemical "sulfonamide") which was used in treatment of Streptococcal Infections. This effort heralded the waves of Antimicrobial Chemotherapy.

Indomethacin (NSAID) was discovered by executing tests on organisms. In vitro concepts were highlighted and the process of synthesis and compound testing came into vogue.

The dawn of understanding approach regarding treatment undertaken was heralded by pioneers namely *Francois Magendie, Claude Beranard* who did few animal experiments to deeply analyse the drug effects. *Rudolf Buchheim* found the first Pharmacology Institute in Germany.

In the dawn of 19th century, *Oswald Schmiedberg* with a brilliant team of *AJ Clark, P Ehrlich, JJ Abel* and many profound students laid the bricks of Fundamentals of pharmacology, no doubt he is known as "The Father of Pharmacology" today!

DRUG DISCOVERY & DRUG INVENTION

Continuous, consistent efforts since those times and still ongoing today have helped us all and thrown a great deal of light to understand mechanism, nature, composition , etc of many drugs.

Ligands are created by enabling 3-D structure Based Drug design (SBDD). Computer Aided Drug Discovery (CADD) , High Throughput screening (HTS) are novel techniques evolving in the 20th century.

DRUG TARGETING

Macromolecules (proteins) are the drug targets which bind to small molecules to treat the diseases.

Small molecules can be Agonists and Antagonists. The former enhance while the latter decrease the influence and final response. Some small molecules can induce irreversible mutations and may serve as Carcinogens. Genomic data availability has led to the advancements in the field of *Proteomics* i.e. study of translational proteins. This has brought forward the knowledge and identification of heightened or depressed protein levels in certain important pathological conditions.

TARGET VALIDATION

Once the drugs are identified as potential candidates, there are sought much thorough and robust evidences which prove the inherent capability of a drug to treat a disease and be useful therapeutically. This process minimises the chances of a drug failing in clinical trials. One of the common procedures is the use of "Chemical probes". Another method is to silence genes by RNA modification. "Knockout mice" and "Transgenic mice" are also great alternatives. In the former, gene coding is totally put off and in the latter promoters guide gene expression.

DRUGGABLE TARGETS

Druggability refers to affinity of the target drug to bind with the small molecule. When the new drug can successfully bind to the small molecule, it is referred to as *first in class.* Such "First In Class" drugs are the final dream destination of every "Drug Discovery" endeavour.

"Me-too-drugs" are the ones which are already validated by a "First-in-class" drug.

Such efforts aim to improve upon the already able "First-in class" drugs which are then turned to novel and better- "Best-in-class" drugs.

POLYPHARMACOLOGY

When target proteins contain similar binding sites, then they serve as targets to many drugs. Hitting many target drugs altogether interrupts the sequential steps in a particular process. There are hints of greater efficacy than hitting a single protein target molecule.

"Systems Pharmacology" is the study of complex molecular systems in relation to drug action.

Adverse effects of Polypharmacology is risk of toxicity.

Binding is influenced not only by "Affinity" but also by "Specificity" of the drug. "Structure" of the target protein containing binding pockets also affects the binding potential of the drug up to a greater extent. The drug must also be able to induce "Allosteric" conformational change to bring about the desired effect.

"Clinical candidate" refers to a drug which binds to the target with great affinity and specificity, produces desired effect and is all in all a safe, efficacious drug.

"Medicinal Chemistry" is the concept of development of new drugs by synthesising and purifying compounds. It also includes drug designing.

HIGH THROUGHPUT SCREENING

In this process automation and robotics are used to test millions of compounds.

Fractions of compound samples drawn from "Chemical library" are placed in multiwell plates for testing. Cautious monitoring of the process should be done to test "hit compounds" against the false positives.

"Structure Activity Relationships" (SAR) and many other properties serve as a guide to finally select the "Lead Compounds" which harbinger the "Lead Optimisation" process.

A "Clinical candidate" is developed with many backup compounds to serve as alternatives in rare events of failure of the Clinical candidate.

"Fragment based Drug discovery" (FBDD) is the process in which big compounds are broken down into their substructures which are tested for suitable small compounds for the target. Later they could be assembled into larger compounds. "Fragment linking" and "Fragment growing" after binding to the desired site on the target can help develop the desired compound by focusing on productive chemical components.

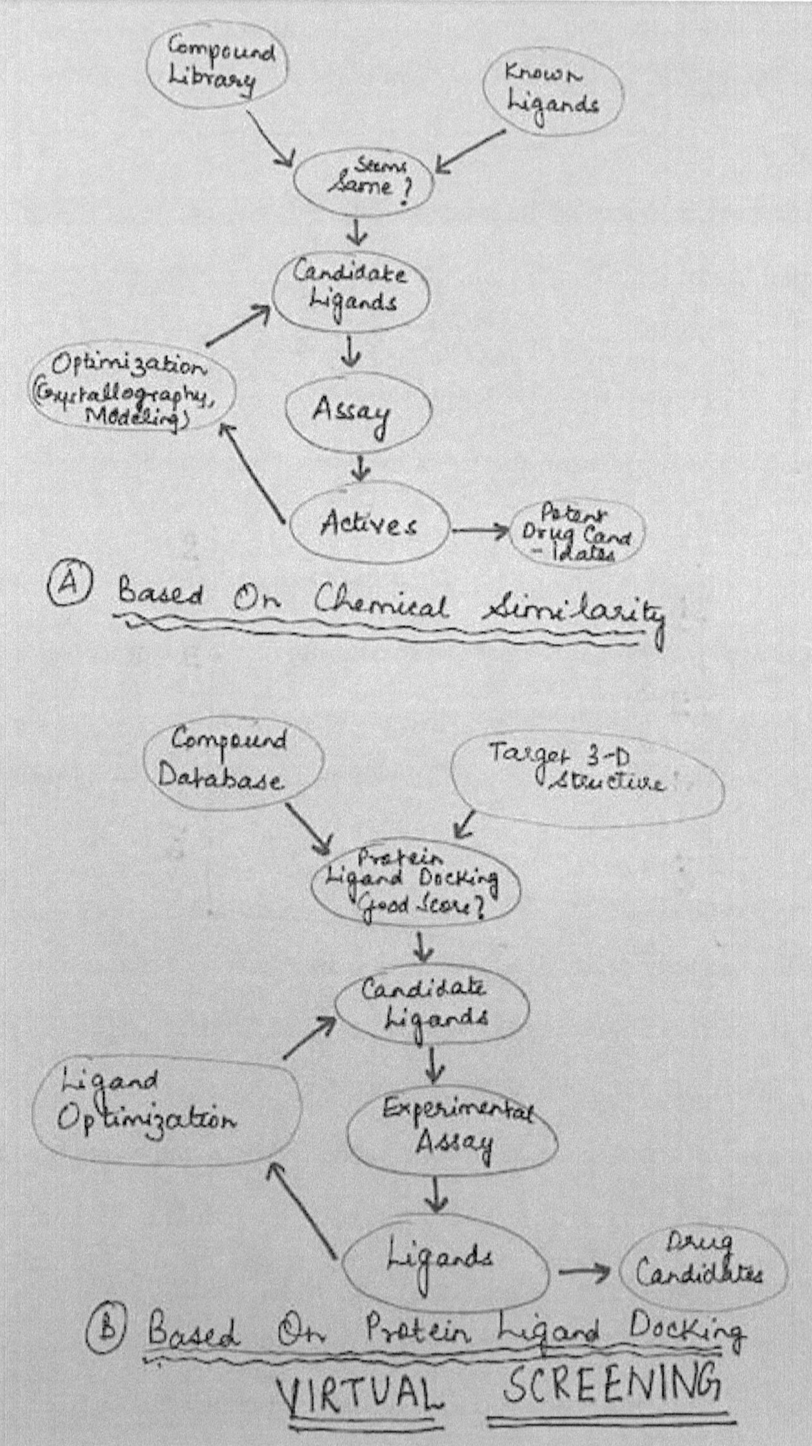

Compound Library
Known Ligands
Seems Same?
Candidate Ligands
Optimization (Crystallography, Modeling)
Assay
Actives
Potent Drug Cand-idates
(A) Based On Chemical Similarity
Compound Database
Target 3-D Structure
Protein Ligand Docking Good Score?
Candidate Ligands
Ligand Optimization
Experimental Assay
Ligands
Drug Candidates
(B) Based On Protein Ligand Docking
VIRTUAL SCREENING

COMPUTER AIDED DRUG DISCOVERY (CADD)

Advancements in Computers and IT have made all the arduous and voluminous tasks easy and possible. Some notable features related to chemical experiments and information are data writing, maintaining, storing, recording and calculating. Computer models are a great aid in drug discovery.

Levels of achievement and accuracy are heightened in the drug discovery process with the computer and technology aids.

Some exceptional achievements are like:

- Discovery of Targeted Ligands

  Chemically similar substrates serve as great harbingers for the drug design process. For already developed drugs, there is greater scope of Me-too-drugs with improved drug profile.

  Various approaches can be molecular fingerprinting, comparison of shapes and electrical fields generated by two different molecules and computation of "Descriptors" like molecular weight, number of aromatic rings, electrical dipole etc. "Virtual screening" could be a quick and affordable alternative to HTS especially when 3-D protein structures of target molecules are not determined.

- Structure Based Drug design

  When 3-D structures of target molecules are known, many more computational methods are known to aid in drug designing. This leads to development of high quality drug targets. By computing atomic forces, atomistic detail simulation can be achieved. Protein ligand binding free energies methods are used to accurately predict protein ligand binding affinities. Variety of conformations adopted by a protein are explored with fast molecular simulation methods. "Molecular Docking" is another alternative to HTS. In this method- the lowest energy and most stable target's binding sites are identified. The calculations are utilised in "Virtual HTS"

AI (ARTIFICIAL INTELLIGENCE) IN DRUG DISCOVERY

Image recognition and Language translation are AI tools much in vogue in the drug discovery process. The existing data guides these tools for accurate prediction of small molecule & protein binding and designing of automated ligands for a targeted protein. 3-D protein structures can too be predicted by using AI tools. Artificial Intelligence holds great prospects in drug discovery in future times.

DRUG DEVELOPMENT

INVESTIGATIONAL NEW DRUG APPLICATION

This is the first step in the Drug Development process. Every sponsor must first and foremost file an Investigational New Drug Application (IND) and submit to FDA to conduct human research with the drug.

- What is IND?

It is the detailed information and basic idea of drug research and investigation in humans. Its elements consist of rationale, evidence of the experimentations which were successfully done, basic pharmacology, adverse reactions info, chemical structural and interaction details and manufacturing info, etc.

Within a month span, the IND is reviewed - can be accepted, improved upon or rejected.

- What is the Role of FDA?

Major responsibility of FDA, the federal regulatory body in the US is to protect and ensure safety, efficacy of all kinds of drugs, medicines, devices for medical use, food supply and products, cosmetics and radiation producing substances.

It also bears responsibility to protect and enhance people's health in general in all possible ways and manners.

It covers not only safety, efficacy, affordability, accessibility of the important drugs, products and food, etc., but its scope is much wider to cover aspects of the toxicity and timely approval of New Drug Application (NDA).

- What are the ethical principles of Clinical Trials?

Before any clinical trial begins, it should satisfy 7 ethical principles:

1. Social & clinical value
2. Scientific validity
3. Fair subjects' selection
4. Informed consent
5. Favourable risk benefit ratio
6. Independent review
7. Respect of potential & enrolled subjects

- What are the phases of Clinical trials?

1. Phase 1
2. Phase 2
3. Phase 3
4. Phase 4

Phases 1-3 are conducted to ensure efficacy and safety while Phase 4 consist of Post marketing trials and collection of information by administering drugs to larger numbers of people and also information about effects, adverse effects, etc.

PHASE 1

- It is done in about 10 to 100 healthy participants (rarely people with severe pathologies are considered).
- It is open label and the main concerns are Safety & Tolerability
- Time taken for this phase is around 1-2 years, it is most inexpensive as compared to other phases and has maximum success rate

PHASE 2

- It is done on 50-500 participants who are patients and are administered the experimental drug.
- It is RCT (Randomised & controlled) mainly, occasionally blinded. The main concerns are efficacy & dose ranging
- Time taken for this phase is around 2-3 years and it's more expensive than Phase 1 trials and success rate is less as compared to Phase 1 trials

PHASE 3

- It is done in a few hundreds to few thousand participants who are patients and are administered the experimental drug.
- It is RCT or uncontrolled, and can be blinded. The main concern is to ensure efficacy in a larger number of people.

- The time taken for this project is 3-5 years and it's very expensive with a very low success rate.

NDA is applied after Phase 3

- It comprises of individual case reports of subjects who were tested
- 6-10 month thorough review process is undertaken
- "Label" (package insert)- the official prescribing info has to be approved

PHASE 4

- It is done in many thousands of people who are receiving treatment with the approved drug.
- It is an open label trial phase. Main concerns are to know adverse effects, various drug interactions, long term effects and patient compliance.
- It's of no fixed duration and the cost or expenses may be variable.

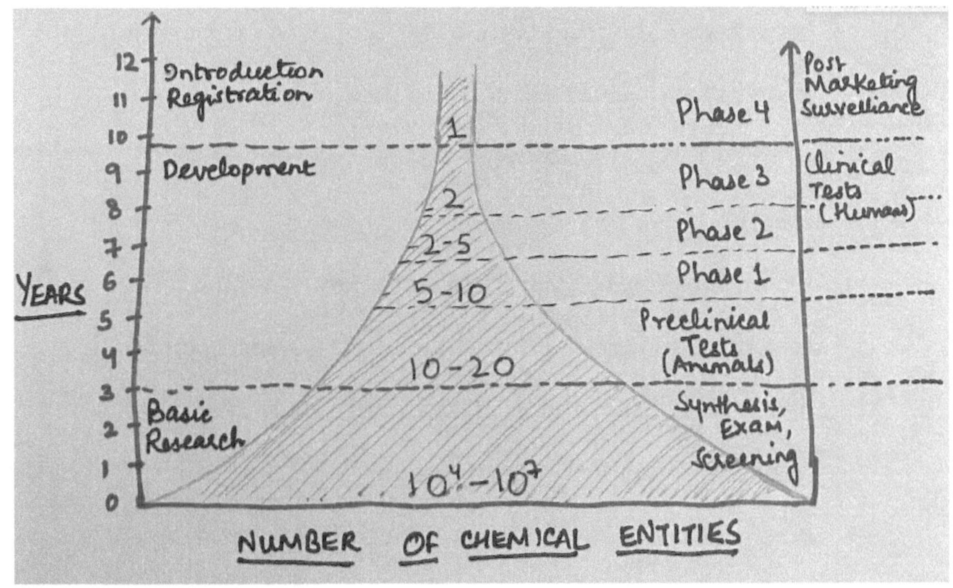

PERSONALISED (INDIVIDUALISED, PRECISION) MEDICINE

- Fitting the drug to Individual patient

- It is due to deep heterogeneity of the person taking drugs and the process of the targeted pathology,

- Great in depth knowledge of genetics and genomics, especially DNA sequencing is a very quick, powerful and affordable method.

- Thorough study of large populations- their medical histories, phenotype characters, diagnostic tests, drug effects, adverse effects and proper follow up provides great insights for this arduous task.

- All such methods help to choose the most appropriate drug. One good example is to choose the most apt drug for cancer chemotherapy i.e. to "HIT" a mutated target when cancer is actively spreading. Similarly, it can be applied to choose most apt patients for specific trials and save time and money.

BIOSIMILARS

- Definition- The biological product is greatly similar to the reference product in terms of safety, purity, efficacy and potency. There must be apt and satisfactory evidence from all kinds of analytics, animal and human studies.

- Need- is for the large molecules especially proteins whose slight modifications in conformation leads to significant pharmacokinetic and pharmacodynamic changes, hence it would be quite tedious to demonstrate equality on therapeutic grounds with the reference product.

ME-TOO DRUGS

- It's a drug or a pharmaceutical very much similar to a drug or medicine already in vogue in the market.

- Some me-too drugs are newly packaged and promoted drugs though similar drugs are available on the market e.g. Esomeprazole and Omeprazole. Such practices distribute the price share.

- Some cons to know are that the Me-too drugs are more expensive. While pros may include better efficacy and less side effects. Some me-too drugs become very popular from a medical point of view and consequently the bestsellers. E.g. Atorvastatin.

CONCLUSION

- There is a need and demand for better and personalised medicine obtained from the latest genetic and molecular diagnostic methods.

- Computational chemistry and computer aided drug designs are integrated with the genetics and molecular biology techniques.

- Present times demand efficacious and more specific treatment techniques for a larger number of people.

Let Us Define

Definitions & terms of high importance and relevance

PHARMACOLOGY:

"Pharmacon"=Drug (in Greek), "Logos"=Science

It is the study of substances that interact with living systems through chemical processes. The substance binds to the regulatory molecules and further may activate or inhibit normal body functions or processes.

A branch of science dealing with mechanism, uses, adverse effects and finally fate of drugs in the body of living beings.

A/ Pharmacology is broadly categorised into:

1. PHARMACODYNAMICS:

   It is the study of all physiological and biochemical drug effects and mechanisms. In short it explains - "What the drug does to the body"

2. PHARMACOKINETICS:

   It is the study of movement of drugs and changes occurring in the drugs inside the body. It encompasses processes like absorption, distribution, metabolism and excretion of drugs, abbreviated as

ADME study. In short it explains, "What the body does to the drugs".

B/ Other miscellaneous branches worth knowing are:

3. MEDICAL PHARMACOLOGY:

   It is the study and science of substances used to prevent, diagnose and treat a disease.

4. PHARMACY:

   It is the science of identifying, compounding, dispensing drugs, forming them into appropriate dosage forms to be easily taken by the patient.

5. PHARMACOTHERAPEUTICS:

   Study to apply combined knowledge of disease and its pharmacological aspect so as to prevent/cure it.

6. PHARMACEUTICS:

   It comprises the manufacture process of drugs and chemicals at large scale.

7. CLINICAL PHARMACOLOGY:

   Study of overall drug profile in all kinds of individuals whether ill or healthy. It also covers safety, drug efficacy, trials, surveys, etc.

8. TOXICOLOGY:

   It is the study of undesirable effects of chemicals on living organisms. We can also define it as the study of different types of toxic conditions of drugs, poisons and poisoning. It also covers the diagnosis and cure of poisoning.

9. CHEMOTHERAPY:

Study of drugs used to prevent or treat diseases caused by microorganisms (infection) and malignancy (cancer).

10. PHARMACOGENETICS:

It is the study of genetic variations in different individuals manifested as differences in drug response or in drug metabolism, mostly they are single gene in origin .E.g. Variations in acetylation phenomenon make an individual either slow or fast acetylator. Former exhibit peripheral neuritis and latter show hepatotoxicity.

11. PHARMACOEPIDEMIOLOGY:

Study of various therapeutic uses, adverse effects of a drug in a defined large (group) population.

C/ Some of the important terms are as follows:

12. DRUG:

"Drogue"=dry herb (in french)

WHO has defined drug as-Any substance or chemical product used or intended to be used to modify or explore physiological system or pathological state for the benefit of the recipient.

13. DRUG COMPENDIA:

Official collections published by the Government body of a country are namely Pharmacopoeias and Formulary. Former are of value to drug producers and contain all details of drugs while the latter in booklet form are of great value to physicians containing information relevant to them like name, dose, indications, side effects, etc.

Non official compendia are Martindale:The complete drug reference (an all-inclusive voluminous publication by Royal Pharmaceutical Society of Great Britain), Merck Index and Physician drug reference (PDR), AMA Drug evaluations (by American Medical Association and Council on Drugs), Modern Encyclopaedia (by Yorke Medical books,USA)

Pharmacopoeia	Formulary
British Pharmacopoeia (BP)	Pharmaceutical Codex(from Pharmaceutical Society Of Great Britain)
United States Pharmacopoeia(USP)	National Formulary (from American Pharmaceutical Association)
Indian Pharmacopoeia (IP)	National Formulary Of India

Table 1. Official Compendia of different regions

14. DRUG CATEGORIES:

There are two major drug categories, first Prescription Drugs which are obtained from the market only after producing a prescription for the drug (Atorvastatin, Levothyroxine, Metformin, Metoprolol). Second category is Non Prescription drugs or better termed as Over the Counter Drugs for which no prescription is required (vitamins, paracetamol, antacids)

15. PROTOTYPE DRUG:

It is a selected drug from a group of drugs chosen to study, pay attention to and demonstrate the most common characteristics, functions and pharmacological effects of that particular group of drugs as a whole. E.g. For local anaesthetics, the prototype drug is Lignocaine.

16. SPURIOUS DRUGS:

If a drug is produced with a name belonging to any other drug, or it is a copy of any other drug, or there is some component little or whole of any other drug, the name of manufacturer is borrowed from any other drug, it is falsely claimed and contaminated , then such drugs are called Spurious drugs.

17. ME-TOO DRUGS:

A drug having very similar structure and only slight differences from another drug then it is called a Me-too drug of another drug. They possess similar mechanisms, indications and side effects. The differences are observed in parameters like t1/2, Vd, E.g. Amitriptyline, Doxepin, Nortriptyline are me-too drugs of Imipramine, Other examples are esketamine, diazepam, etc.

18. ESSENTIAL DRUGS:

Drugs serving to fulfil the priority healthcare needs of a population are called Essential Drugs. The important criteria of selection are Disease Incidence and Prevalence, cost effectiveness, quality assurance, safety and efficacy of drug. WHO brought out the first list in 1977, since then it is updated every 2 years. Currently, there is an 18th list of medicines and 4th list for childrens' medicine by WHO updated in 2013. In India, the first list was out in 1996, Currently it was revised in 2013, it contains 406 medicines.

19. ORPHAN DRUGS:

These are medicines or products to prevent or treat some rare disease or condition. It is assumed that sales of drugs are meagre and cannot make up for their production cost.(Haem arginate used to treat acute intermittent porphyria). The Orphan Drug Act of 1983 has clearly stated about the rare disease as, "Any disease/condition which affects less than two lac individuals (in USA) or more than two lac individuals for whom there is no expectation of recovery of cost of developing and making in the USA is known as rare disease and drugs used to treat these states are known as Orphan drugs". Till date up to 300 orphan drugs have been approved by FDA for more than 82 rare diseases discovered.

Nature and Sources Of Drugs

Drugs can be:

- Simple or complex

- Organic or inorganic

- Acidic or basic

- Solid or liquid or gaseous

- Small or large

Drug Sources:

1. Plants-

- Medicinal plants like opium, ephedra, cinchona, belladonna, foxglove, etc have been derived and adopted from different systems all round the world.

- Different ingredients are Alkaloids (morphine, nicotine, quinine, ephedrine, reserpine, etc), Glycosides (cardiac like digoxin, strophanthin, aminoglycosides like gentamicin) are made of combined sugar and non sugar moiety, Oils may be fixed (groundnut oil, sesame oil, castor oil) or essential (peppermint oil, eucalyptus oil, clove oil) made from plant material serve as carminatives, flavoring agents. Liquid paraffin, hard paraffin are obtained from minerals.

- Tannins , Astringents, Gums, Demulcents, vehicles , suspending agents

2. Animals-

Both animal parts and organ extracts are used to develop important drugs like adrenaline, insulin, vaccines, antiser etc.

3. Minerals-

Iodine, Lithium salts, aluminium and magnesium salts are used for therapeutic purposes.

4. Microbes-

Medicines like tetracyclines, penicillins, streptomycin(Antibiotics) are obtained from microorganisms. Some enzymes (diastase) and vaccines are also developed in similar manner.

5. Synthetic drugs-

Presently, it's the biggest medicinal production unit. It has people's faith and support due to services like purification of products and getting the desired number of medicines. Variety of analogues , congeners, forms of drugs can be manufactured giving priority to new, selective drug effects. (ACE Inhibitors, HIV reverse transcriptase inhibitors, fluoroquinolones, thiazides, etc.) There are many advantages of synthetic sources of drugs as compared to natural sources:

- Proper quality control can be achieved.

- The process becomes easy and less expensive

- Modification in product's chemical structure and physical properties can be done for betterment, more safety and potency.

6. Biologic Agents/ Biopharmaceutical agents/ Recombinant DNA Technology

Genetic Engineering is a very potent tool in which genetic material is manipulated, desired genes are inserted in different bacterial strains e.g. E.Coli K 12, which becomes capable of producing certain proteins away from normal course. It is today much in vogue, new customised products/drugs can be made (monoclonal antibodies, human insulin, growth hormones and growth factors) all to make drugs a better entity to achieve desired therapeutic results. E.g. Humulin (human insulin) and Recombivax-HB (Hepatitis -B vaccine).

Name Of Drugs

Mainly three types of drug names are significant to know:

1. Chemical name-

   This is the chemical structure name of the drug or medicine, and hence is difficult to remember and to be used, so avoided in prescribing.

2. Non proprietary name or Generic name-

   This is the name accepted by a competent authority like British Approved Name (BAN) or United States Approved Name (USAN) .These names are kept unchanged in WHO member countries simply by an agreement rINN (Recommended International Non proprietary name). Later these enter the pharmacopoeia and become official names!

3. Proprietary name or Brand name-

   This is the name coined by the manufacturer and hence is his trademark name. Quality of these names is they are quite easy to recall and remember but they are specific for a region many a times and their name is changing from place to place, manufacturer to manufacturer.

Chemical Name	Non Proprietary name	Proprietary name
Acetyl Salicylic Acid	Aspirin	Ecosprin (USV, India) Mejoral (CFL Pharma Ltd, India) Disprin (Rickett and Benckiser India)
Aminobenzyl penicillin	Ampicillin	Biocillin (Biochem Pharma , India) Roscillin (Ranbaxy, india) Albercillin (Aventis, India)

Table 2. Drug examples with 3 types of names

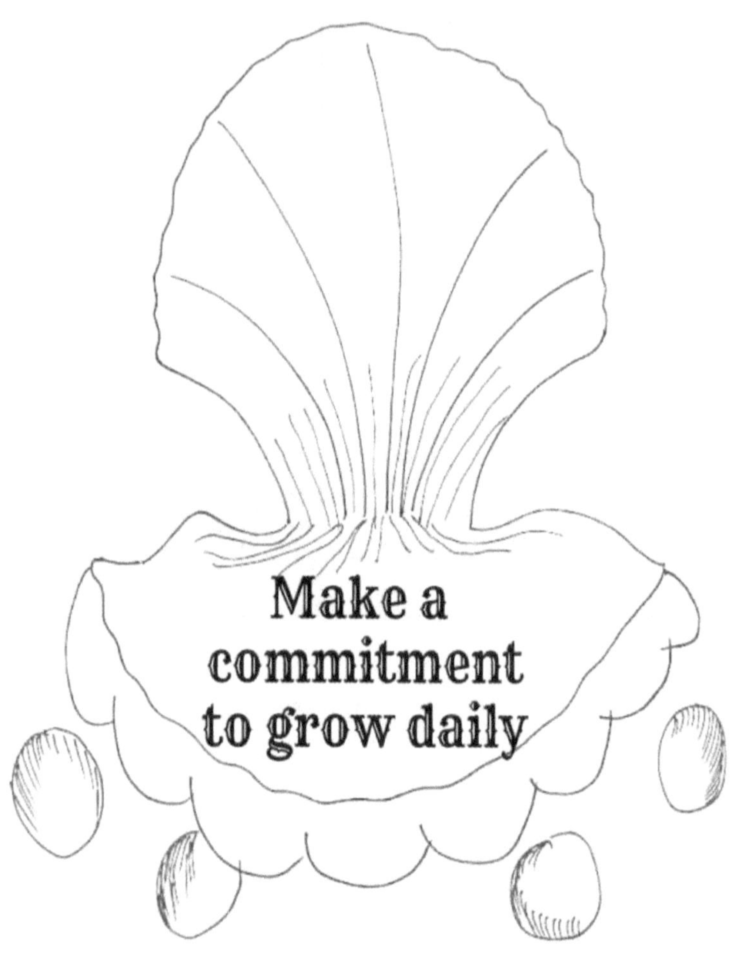

Make a
commitment
to grow daily

Chapter 2

Pharmacokinetics at a Glance-1

KEY FEATURES

- *Introduction to Pharmacokinetics*
- *Basics of Membrane Transport*
- *Routes of Drug Administration*
- *Dosage Forms of Drugs*
- *Drug Absorption*
- *Drug Distribution*
- *Drug Biotransformation*

Definition:

The quantitative study governing the complete motion of drugs in the body, through the body, outside the body is termed as Pharmacokinetics. All the key processes in this regard like Absorption , Distribution, Metabolism and Excretion of drugs are a part of this study , hence this is also termed as "ADME" study.

This study forms the basis to determine dose of drug, routes of drug administration, duration and frequency of drug action.

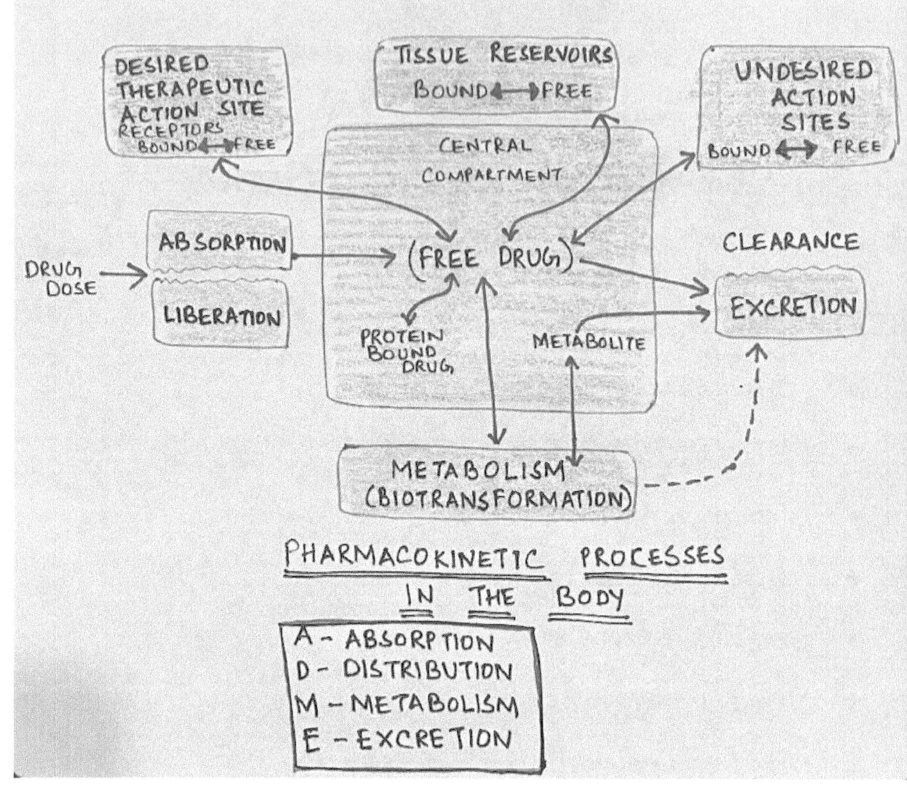

Fig 3. Various Pharmacokinetic processes in the body

Basics of Membrane Transport:

A biological membrane is a double layer composed of cholesterol and phospholipids. Drug movement and transport across this membrane happens by mainly following processes:

1. Passive diffusion:

   Diffusion of drugs occurs across membranes in direction from high to low concentration gradient. It is the most common mechanism for all drugs. When a drug is highly lipid soluble, it easily achieves a good concentration in the membranes, and the process hastens, rate of transport is directly proportional to the lipid:water partition coefficient.

Henderson Hasselbalch Equation: pH Influence:

Log [Protonated form]/[unprotonated form]

=pKa-pH

Ionisation of weak acids and weak basic drugs is pH dependent. Strong acids and strong basic drugs remain ionised in all ranges of pH.

Weak acid Ionisation is described the formula:

$$pH = pKa + \log (A^-/HA)$$

Here, if value of (A^-/HA) is equal to one, then log 1=0, therefore:

$$pH = pKa$$

Hence we infer following:

- pKa is equal to pH at which drug is 50% ionised.

- Weak acid drugs form salts (sodium sulfadiazine, sodium phenobarbitone) and ionise more at alkaline pH.

- Weak bases form salts (atropine sulphate, ephedrine hydrochloride) and ionise more at acidic pH.

- Acidic drugs ionise more in alkaline urine and are excreted fast, while oppositely, basic drugs ionise more in acidic urine and excreted fast.

As described, there occurs a relationship amongst the pH of the medium , dissociation constant of the drug (pKa) and degree of ionisation.

This whole concept is defined and equated by Henderson Hasselbalch equation:

pKA(Acid) = pH + log {Concentration of Non Ionised Acid/Concentration Of Ionised Acid}

pKA(Base) = pH + log {Concentration of Ionised Base/Concentration Of Non Ionised Base}

We infer from above equation the following:

- If the acid is strong or the base is weak, it will decrease its pKa and vice versa.
- When pKa of a drug= pH of the medium, the drug will be half (50%) ionised and half (50%) non ionised.
- If the pH of the drug and the surrounding medium is the same, drugs are readily absorbed. E.g. Weakly acidic drugs like barbiturates, aspirin etc. are non ionised in stomach acidic medium and their absorption is favoured. Weakly basic drugs like morphine, diazepam , etc. are non ionised in intestinal alkaline pH and there they are highly absorbed.
- In case of one unit shift in pH (increase or decrease), there occurs 10 unit similar change(increase or decrease respectively) in degree of ionised and non ionised drug fraction (weak acid or weak base)
- Some types of drugs, like strongly basic or strongly acidic as a rule -"Always stay ionised at all pH values", so their absorption suffers greatly.

Ion Trapping:

When acidic drugs are in unionised state in the stomach, they easily cross the gastric mucosal membrane, and once inside, they convert to ionised form as pH is little high (pH=7.0) and then it becomes impossible for them to pass on further, so with slow speed, they enter ECF. This whole process is known as *"Ion Trapping"*. So you can imagine, if the drug is Aspirin, it will get trapped and cause a lot of destruction to gastric mucosal cells. Plant hormones subjected to this process are Abscisic acid and Retinoic acid. Animal hormones subjected to this process are prostacyclins and Leukotrienes.

2. Filtration:

Drug passes through membranes via large paracellular spaces (as in capillaries) . This process is hastened by a strong push flow of solvent under hydrostatic or osmotic pressure. In case of capillaries, the diffusion process depends on blood flow rate and not on pH of medium or lipid solubility of drugs.

3. Specialised Transport:

It can be described in following heads:

(a) Carrier Transport:

Almost all types of cell membranes possess a variety of protein molecules which serve as transporters for different ions, transmitters, nutrients and xenobiotics (a substance foreign to the body, not naturally produced or found in the body) . The simple mechanism is that conformational change occurs in the transporters after binding to the substrate which is carried to the destination. Then the substrate is dissociated and transporters regain original shape and form. Various features of this type of transport are- its saturable, substrate specific and can be competitively inhibited. Genetic polymorphism can change both concentration and binding ability of transporter protein overall affecting its pharmacokinetics.

Its two types are:

- Facilitated diffusion- SLC (solute carrier transporters) transporters passively carry substrate in the direction of concentration gradient without utilising any energy.E.g. Transport of glucose and Amino acid into the cell and transport of oxygen into blood and muscles.

- Active Transport- This process requires energy, occurs opposite the concentration gradient, it can be restricted by metabolic poisons and results in deposition of drug at a membrane side.E.g. P-glycoprotein is a non selective transporter aiding in carrying xenobiotics, calcium ions moving from cardiac muscle cells, sodium potassium pump operating in the body and Amino acids moving along intestinal tract. Depending upon source of energy, we can classify active transport as follows:

  ★ Primary active transport- Hydrolysis of ATP is the source of energy. The process involves ATP binding cassette (ABC) transporters which possess ATPase activity in their internal loop sites.

NOTE -P glycoprotein (P-gp) is a famous primary active transporter found mainly in intestine, kidney tubules, around brain capillaries, etc.It performa main function to pump out xenobiotics (foreign substances/drugs) . Other similar transporters are MRP 2 (Multidrug resistance associated protein 2) and BCRP (Breast cancer resistance protein)

★ Secondary Active transport-In this type source of energy to carry one substrate is obtained by downhill movement of another substrate. The process involves SLC transporters which perform both uptake and efflux functions. E.g. Cocaine, SSRIs utilise SERT, NET,etc. which are active SLC transporters, Glucose is absorbed in intestines and kidney. via SGLT1 and SGLT2 which are also secondary active transporters.

Co transport or Symport is a term used to describe movement of both substrates in the same direction.

Exchange transport or Antiport is a term used to describe movement of substrates in different directions.

NOTE- Organic anion transporting polypeptide (OATP) and Organic cation transporter (OCT) are famous examples of Secondary active transporters found in liver and kidney.

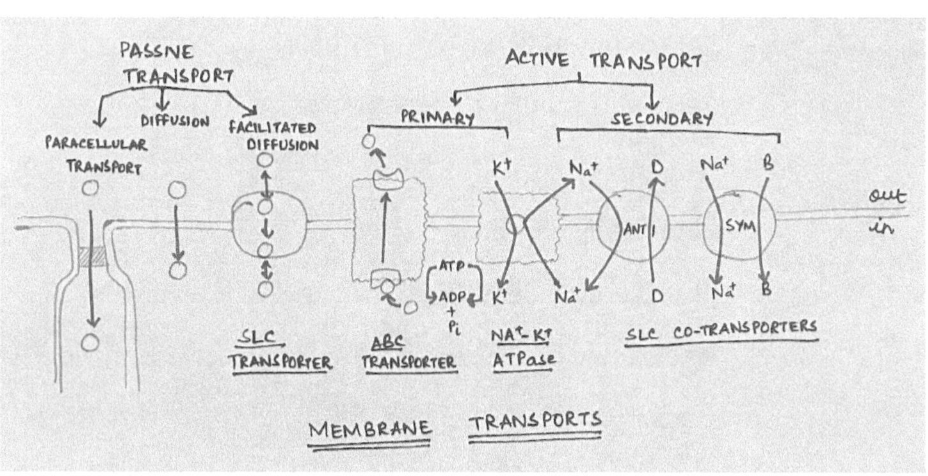

(b) Vesicular Transport:

Movement of large impermeable particles, substances inside and outside of cells by formation of vesicles bound by inclusion of cell membrane is generally termed as Vesicular transport. When enclosed particles are moved in , it's called *"Endocytosis"* and when moved out, it's called *"Exocytosis"*. In detail, a binding protein on a cell membrane forms a complex with the particle to stimulate formation of the vesicle, after complete enclosure, the vesicle detaches from the cell to carry the large molecule or particle. E.g. Stimulation of nerve cells occurs to make storage vesicles reach the surface and extrude out stored neurotransmitters like Nor Adrenaline. Secretion of Insulin is another classic example.

Let us brief out Endocytosis:

Exogenous molecules are taken up inside plasma membrane derived vesicles. The process can be of two major types:

- Pinocytosis (Fluid uptake)- *"Pino"= I drink* (Greek), *"Cytos"= hollow vessel*
  In this, fluid or solution of drugs is taken inside.
  E.g. Insulin moves across BBB via this process and

Liposomes of Antitumor drugs are biotransported also through this process. The process marks importance for small quantities of drugs, occurs mainly at lung alveoli and blood vessel wall.

- Phagocytosis (particle uptake)- *"phago"=to eat* It's a rare procedure in which the particulate molecules or substances are transferred in vesicles formed by membranous invaginations. Certain amount of energy is also required in the process. E.g. Antigen ingestion leads to allergic reactions and botulinum toxin poisoning utilises this process as an absorptive procedure.

Routes Of Drug Administration

There are a variety of routes of drug administration. There are some important criteria to judge and choose a certain route. The main ones to list are:

1. Drug Properties- Physical (solid/liquid/gas) and Chemical (pH, solubility, etc.)
2. Desired site of action- Feasible or non feasible and Local or General
3. Rate of absorption of a drug and its extent upto which it gets absorbed.
4. First pass metabolism effect on drug
5. Desired speed of action of drug
6. Patient state (co-operative or non co-operative)

Routes of Drug Administration

Flowchart

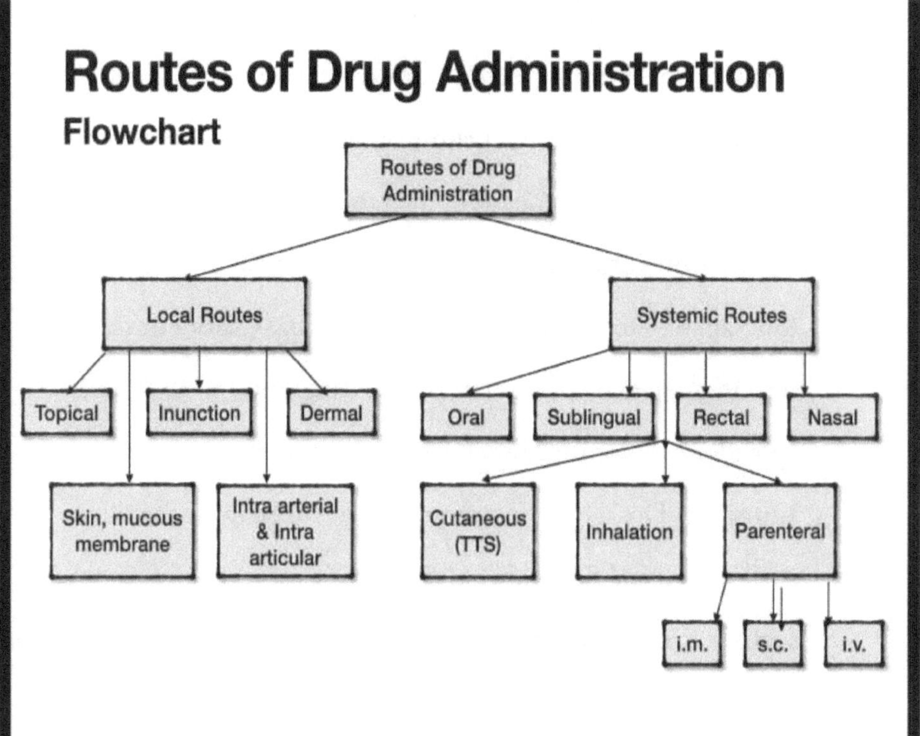

Mainly there are two heads under which we can classify these routes:

A/ Local routes:

These are the preferred sites of drug action when systemic effect can be minimal or not desired at all. Specificity of drug action is achieved and satisfactory results are seen with a good amount of drug at desired site.

Local routes are as follows:

1. Topical:

    Drugs are applied externally, they easily show desired results at specific sites with almost nil systemic effects. Desired sites can be skin, ear, eye, nasal mucosa, anal canal, vagina, etc. Different dosage forms for this purpose are external (dusting) powders, lotions, ointments, gels, creams, suppositories, pessaries. Apart from these, some more sites and dosage forms are included in this route. Drugs given orally for local action in GIT (Sucralfate, vancomycin), Inhalational drugs (Salbutamol, terbutaline), and Urethral irrigation drugs in form of *Bougies* (povidone iodine) are also a part of this route.

Inunction Dosage forms are applied by rubbing on the skin surface. Dermal drugs are either dusted or sprayed over the skin surface. Both forms are safe and easy to administer. E.g. Antibiotic ointments, powders and solutions are used for local effects like antipruritic, antifungal and analgesic. Antiseptic powders are dusted and analgesic sprays are widely used.

2. Intra-arterial and Intra-articular routes:

    Sometimes drugs are injected little deep with no systemic effect desired as in intra-articular injection (hydrocortisone acetate), nerve infiltration and intrathecal injection (lidocaine).

    Accurate intra arterial injection is applied to introduce contrast media in angiography and to administer anticancer drugs to treat leg malignant states.

B/ Systemic routes

The basic motto to use these routes is to have a systemic effect of drugs. Absorption via circulation occurs for drugs through these routes.

1. Oral:

    This is the most easy, common, cheap and traditional method of taking drugs. Solid dosage forms (powders, tablets, capsules, pills) as well as liquid dosage forms (syrups, linctus, elixirs) can be taken via this route.

    Variable absorption trend, slow action, propensity to be degraded by stomach HCl and inappropriateness for non tasty drugs, non co-operative patients makes this route selective to a little extent.

2. Sublingual route:

    In this route, drug is placed under the tongue, where it gets dissolved and absorbed quickly in circulation. It is suitable for lipid soluble medicines and once the effect is achieved, leftover drug should be spitted out of the mouth. Though a little tricky and inconvenient, it has a great benefit of bypassing first pass metabolism and hence bioavailability of drugs is increased.

3. Cutaneous: Transdermal Therapeutic system (TTS)

    When a drug is highly lipid soluble and is applied on the skin surface, it slowly percolates through a cutaneous route and is absorbed for a long duration. Transdermal therapeutic preparations are simply adhesive occlusive patches through which drug travels at a constant rate via the skin layers and enters the blood circulation. There is a drug reservoir in between the backing plate and controlled drug release membrane, it gets attached via adhesive film to the skin surface (contains an initial concentrated drug form). Drug entry is via a diffusion mechanism. Preferred sites for such drug delivery routes are on the chest, abdomen, back, upper arm, hips, etc. Drugs administered via this route are Glyceryl trinitrate (GTN), nicotine, fentanyl, hyoscine, clonidine, etc.

Advantages of this type of drug delivery route are convenience and preference over oral route as they show less side effects. High cost and local irritation rarely are observed drawbacks.

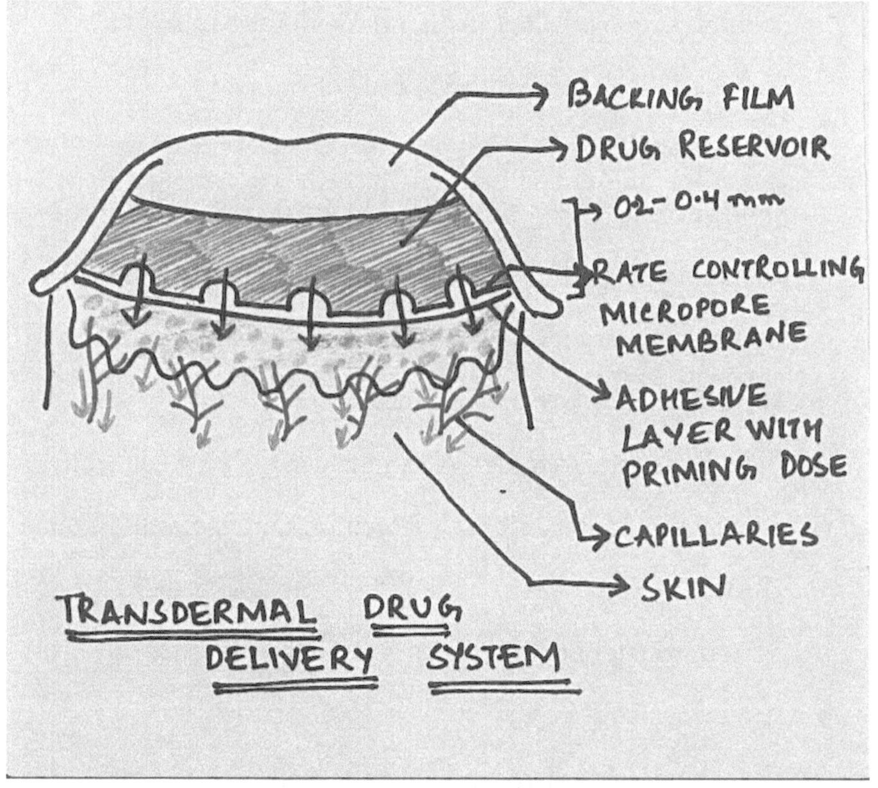

Fig 1. Transdermal Drug Delivery System

4. Nasal:

Drugs like calcitonin, GnRH agonists, desmopressin are given via this route in the form of spray, etc. Advantages are that this route bypasses first pass metabolism and drugs are easily absorbed.

5. Inhalation:

Drugs given via this route for systemic action are mainly General anaesthetics. Rapid drug absorption takes place from a large area of lung alveoli. When desired effect is achieved, drug administration is halted and it quickly diffuses back. Only drawback is lung irritation and inflammation.

6. Parenteral routes:

It is the route "par" "enterum", i.e. away from the intestine. In this the drug is administered through injection at various sites so as to bypass first pass metabolism and achieve quick, site specific and accurate results. Generally no incidences of nausea, gastric disturbances are seen. Drawbacks include high cost, difficult, painful procedures and rarely lacerations of surrounding skin or tissue.

Various routes under this head are as follows:

- Intramuscular (i.m.):

Drug is injected in large skeletal muscles like the arm (deltoid), upper outer posterior buttock (gluteus maximus), thigh (vastus lateralis), lateral hip (gluteus medius). These sites have great circulation and nerves too. The procedure is painless and contraindicated in patients taking anticoagulant drugs due to risk of hematoma. Depot preparations can be given via this route.

- Intravenous(i.v.):

Drug is either slowly infused over a long duration or can be given as a bolus form. Drug directly enters blood circulation and bypasses the liver, there is 100% bioavailability. Titration of drug dose with response can be easily monitored. Drawbacks observed are Extravasation leading to necrosis of surrounding tissue, thrombophlebitis of vein and air embolism may also be seen.

- Subcutaneous (s.c.):

Drug is injected in the subcutaneous region of the skin. Less volumes are injected. Absorption is seen a little late, so this route is not appropriate for emergency states like shock. *Dermojet* is a needleless system of injection, drug is injected in jet form with high velocity and hence its a painless procedure. *Pellet* is a solid form of drug (DOCA, Testosterone) introduced for drug release over a long duration of time. *Implants* of drugs (hormones, contraceptives) are used to be placed under the skin which release drugs at controlled rate. These implants can be degradable or non biodegradable.

- Intradermal:

A bleb is raised or multiple punctures of skin epidermis is done to inject drugs via this route. It's not a common route. E.g. BCG vaccine is given via this route.

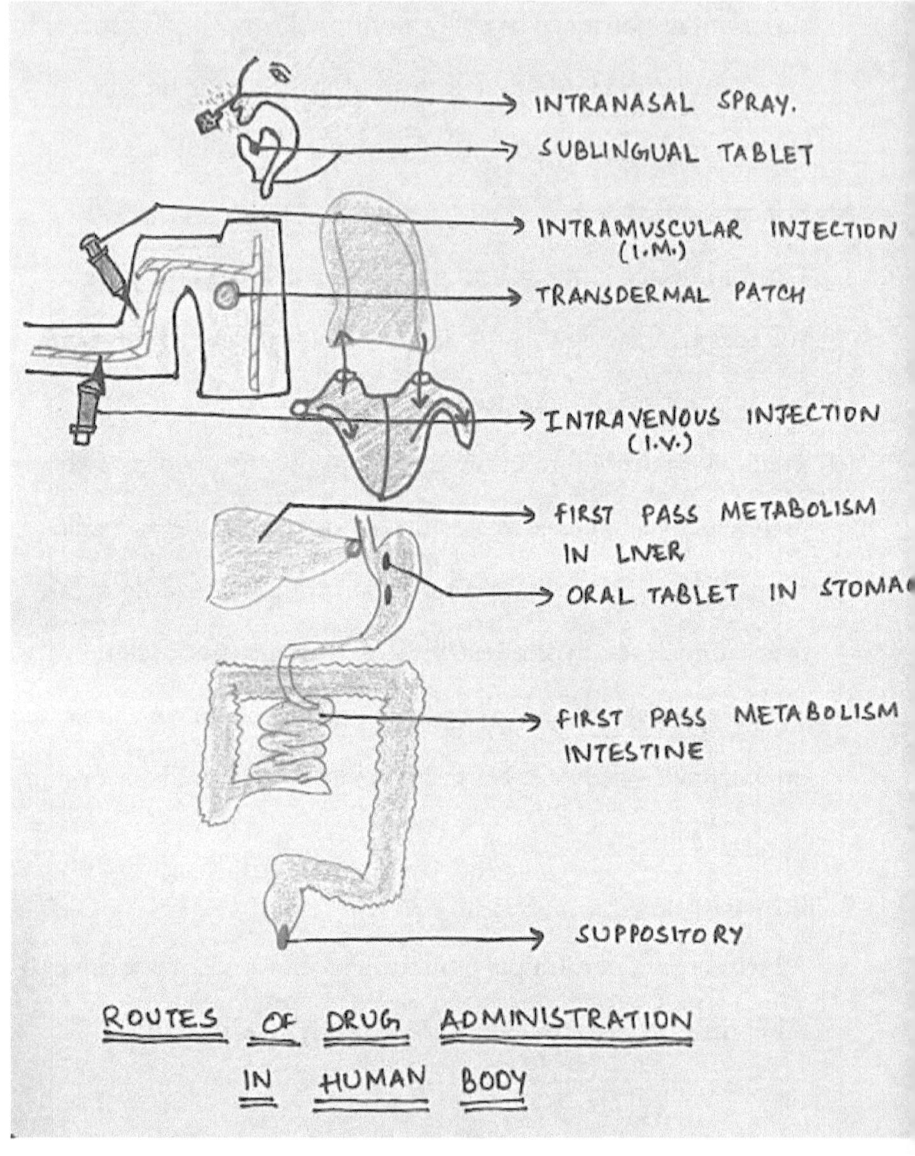

Fig 2. Different Routes of Drug Administration in human body

Dosage Forms of Drugs

Drug dose:

A specific amount of medication taken at one time . These are generally expressed in conventional metric mass units (milligrams, grams, etc.). Few drugs like insulin, heparin are mixture forms having no specific units.

Drug Dosage:

A prescribed administration of a specific amount, number and frequency of doses over a specified time duration.

Formulation:

A recipe to prepare a drug. It is the list of all ingredients like main drug (base), add on drugs (additives), excipients, vehicles, coloring and flavoring agents, etc.

Dosage form:

In this, the active moiety is added upon with necessary additives, excipients, diluents, vehicle etc, i.e. the whole formulation is made up into a dispensable form like packet or bottle (tablet, capsule, suspension, mixture), for convenient administration to the patient.

Dosage forms are of following types

A/ Solid dosage forms

B/ Liquid dosage forms

C/ Semisolid dosage forms

D/ Inhalation dosage forms

E/ Parenteral forms

A/ SOLID DOSAGE FORMS:

1. Powders:

   The finest pulverised form of a drug in dry state is called Powder. It may be for Oral administration or Topical administration.The latter are also referred to as the *Dusting powders.* If the quantity is very large, it is known as *Bulk powders.* Some powders containing soda bicarb salt when dissolved in water, liberate CO_2 producing bubbles, such are known as *Effervescent powders.*

2. Tablets:

   The powder drug form when combined with different substances like additives, binding agents, excipients, diluents, preservatives, etc and shaped into a definite round or elliptical form by compression technique feasible for oral administration, this is called Tablet.

   It can be of many types like Chewable tablets, Dispersible tablet (quickly dispersed in water), Plain tablets (no coating), Enteric coated tablet (it is unaffected by stomach acid and disintegrates only in duodenum), Sugar and film coated tablet (easy and pleasant to be swallowed), Sublingual tablets (taken by putting under the tongue, quickly dissolves in mouth),

Sustained/Extended Release Tablets (Coated with drug particles which disintegrate and dissolve at different time rates and interval, so that longer duration and site specific action can be achieved), Controlled release tablets (drug is slowly released via a membrane).

3. Capsules:

Cylindrical gelatin holders filled with drug particles or drug in gel or liquid form, easily dissolved in water and meant for oral administration. Their types can be Hard gelatin capsules (composed of gelatin, water and also contain sometimes titanium dioxide) , Soft gelatin capsule (same as hard gelatin capsule but moisture proportion differs, plasticizers like Glycerol is added to keep the capsule elastic and stable), HPMC Capsule (contains hydroxypropylmethyl cellulose with water), Pullulan capsule (composed of water soluble mucopolysaccharide , the Pullulan along with water, though water content is very low and quite tough capsules), Enteric coated Capsules (they disintegrate on reaching the ileum and saved from stomach acid), Spansules (contain drug particles coated in layers so that they dissolve at different time periods to make an extended release capsule form)

4. Lozenges:

Drugs along with gum packed and shaped in different forms. They may also contain added sweeteners and flavours. They are kept in

mouth and get slowly dissolved to release the drug for local action
(on throat, etc).

5. Pills:

    Drugs in small round or oval mass meant to be swallowed orally.
    Generally mixed up with sugar syrup or honey to form a small oval
    sticky mass.

6. Suppositories:

    A conical solid form contains medicine, glycerine etc which when
    placed in body orifice or cavity like rectum, urethra or vagina,
    easily melts at body temperature to release the drug which gets
    absorbed in circulation. *Pessaries* are for vaginal administration
    while *Bougies* are long cones meant for urethral administration .

B/ LIQUID DOSAGE FORMS:

1. Solutions:

    Drug is dissolved in water acting as the vehicle meant for oral,
    topical and sometimes parenteral use. It may also contain
    sweeteners, flavours and preservatives.

2. Suspensions:

    Suspending agents (bentonite, tragacanth, kaolin,
    carboxymethylcellulose sodium) are used to help in dispersion of
    insoluble drug particles evenly in the medium or vehicle.

Mixtures are aqueous suspensions in which solid drugs are dispersed homogeneously in aqueous vehicle via a suspending agent , E.g. Milk of Magnesia, Antidiarrhoeal mixtures

Emulsions are suspensions or mixtures of two immiscible liquids (oil and water). Dispersed phase (particles of one liquid) stay suspended in continuous phase (particles of other liquid) with aid of emulsifying agents (agar, albumin, alginate, casein, gum, Irish moss, lecithin, soaps) . Always *"Shake well before Use"*. Milk is a naturally occurring emulsion.

3. Drops:

    Concentrated drug forms as liquid preparations meant for oral and topical (eye drops, ear drops, nose drops) administration.

4. Lotions and Liniments:

    Lotions are solutions or mixtures applied topically on skin without rubbing. They perform functions of soothing, cooling and protecting skin surface from foreign dust, pollution, abrasions, etc. *Liniments* are applied with rubbing and contain *counterirritant* (an agent applied to one part produces irritation in that part and relieves pain or irritation in other body part, mechanism being chemical stimulation of thermal skin receptors, e.g. menthol, wintergreen, eucalyptus, camphor) and are *rubefacient* (a substance when applied on skin produces redness due to capillary dilatation and increase in blood circulation, e.g.

salicylates like Methyl salicylate, Capsaicin derived from chilli pepper) too.

5. Alcoholic Solutions:

    - Elixirs:

      They are hydro alcoholic drug solutions with added sweeteners or flavours. The base is either sugar syrup or glycerol with high alcohol concentrations. E.g. cough elixir, vit B-complex elixir.

    - Spirits:

      Their composition is 10% v/v essential oils (volatile) and alcohol and utilised as flavouring and masking agents. E.g. Spirit chloroform, Spirit ammonium aromaticus.

    - Tinctures:

      These contain plant drugs in composition of 10-20 %, found as extracts of alcohol and are used as flavouring agents . E.g. Tincture cardamom compound , Tr. Zingiberis.

      Another hydroalcoholic composition of inorganic substances is also referred to as Tinctures and finds use as antiseptic , E.g. Tr. Iodine

6. *Linctus* is a viscous solution especially containing menthol (provides cooling sensation) and antitussive (cough suppressants) , meant to be slowly taken for throat ailments.

Syrups contain high sugar and have thick consistency.

C/ SEMI SOLID DOSAGE FORMS:

1. Ointments:

   These are drug preparations in oily bases (hard paraffin, soft paraffin, bee's wax, wool fat) applied topically on dry abrasions or wounds.

2. Pastes:

   These are preparations of finely powdered solids like starch, zinc oxide, calcium carbonate, etc. These compounds absorb water and swell. Pastes are non oily substances containing glycerol, mucilage, soaps, etc. They are applied topically on wet wounds, where they serve to absorb harmful chemicals released by bacteria and wound exudates. Examples are starch paste, mustard, putty, toothpaste, etc.

3. Gels:

   These are viscous semi solid colloids systems in which solid disperse phase forms a network in combination with liquid continuous phase. These dosage forms help in optimum and long lasting cutaneous and percutaneous drug delivery. Curd, cheese and butter are natural gels. Therapeutic gels are aluminium hydroxide gel, aluminium phosphate gel, etc.

4. Creams:

These are of ointment composition but water in oil emulsion. They are less greasy, have better compliance, better absorbed from the skin and used for cosmetic purposes too.

5. Plaster:

It is prepared by mixing a drug in a resinous base, it can be spread over a muslin cloth or coated with water resistant coatings. Their consistency changes from hard at room temperature to sticky at body temperature. Action is protective and antiseptic in nature . E.g. Band- aid, Zinc oxide plaster.

D/ INHALATION DOSAGE FORMS

1. Aerosols:

Aerosols refer to fine mist of spray under pressure systems. These are products of therapeutically active substances packed under pressure, and these can be released upon activation of the proper valve system. The particle size should be controlled, generally kept under 5 micrometres.

2. Nebuliser:

It is a drug delivery device which administers medication as inhaled mist form of the drug into the lungs. There are different types of nebulisers like Pneumatic (Jet nebulisers), Mechanical (Soft mist inhaler), Electrical (Ultrasonic wave nebuliser and

Vibrating mesh technology). Most commonly used are jet nebulisers, also known as *Atomizers*.Compressed gas flows at high velocity through liquid medicament via tubing and converts into mist of air to be inhaled by the patient.

3. Metered Dose Inhaler:

    It is an inhaler device with specified doses and provides a fixed amount of active ingredient dose in each puff.

    Hydrofluoroalkanes are preferred propellants in MDI, pressurised MDI (PMDI) are easy to hold devices which work on principle of pressurised propellant in aerosol chamber. Currently these are prioritised by physicians in prescriptions . Advantages of MDI are accurate and repeatable dosing with least or no error

4. Rotahaler:

    It is an easy to carry device. There is a capsule (Rotacap) which holds very fine drug powder, the capsule is punctured during use by twisting the rotahaler device, which is a two part mouthpiece and released particles are aerosolized by inspiratory flow of the patient.

5. Spinhaler:

    It is also a dry powder inhaler like Rotahaler , the difference being that it consists of three pieces, not two. The pieces are the mouthpiece, tiny fan and a cap to cover the fan, the capsule is put in the fan area, the cap put back and the capsule is crushed. Then the patient tilts head back, puts the mouthpiece in mouth and inhales. The fan throws the medicine into the throat. It is available in the market in small bottle shaped containers, the lid is shaky, not tight while Rotahaler is available in a small compact plastic case with lid intact, and can be easily carried.

E/ PARENTERAL DOSAGE FORMS

1. Injection:

   These are sterile solutions in water or oily vehicles. Then administration is parenteral , via subcutaneous (into fat layer between skin and muscle), intramuscular (deep into muscle) routes. But oily suspensions are not given intravenously (through a vein) as they may lead to hazardous embolism. Injections are called "shot" in the US and "jab" in the UK. The drug is injected into a person's body via needle syringe.

2. Infusion:

   Infusion therapy is used to put large volumes of liquid medicines in a person's body through a needle or catheter. It is a good alternative method when oral therapy is not suitable. It allows for controlled dosing.Along with a lot of drugs especially antibiotics and normal saline, infusion can be used to deliver nutrition too. Infusion bottles available in the market are made of glass or polypropylene.

3. Vial:

   A small cylindrical container made to hold liquid medicines is a Vial. These can be single or multi-dose. Nowadays there are dry powder vials too, in which sterile solvent is mixed just before administration. They are protected by air tight rubber caps.

4. Ampoules:

   These are single doses containing sealed glass containers and broken to be used, hence cannot be used more than once. They are for use and throw purpose, the liquid medication is sucked or drawn via an injection.

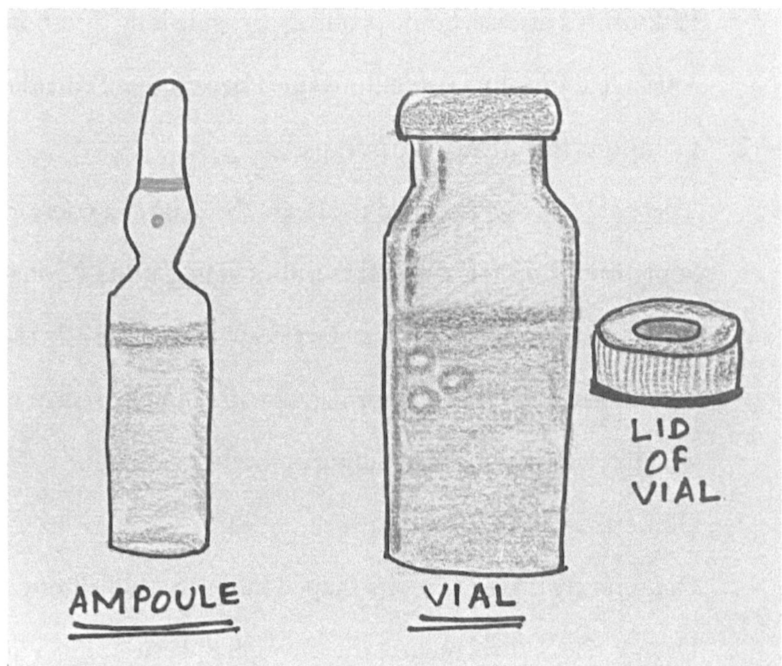

F/ TARGETING OF DRUGS: SPECIAL DRUG DELIVERY SYSTEMS

Purpose of Targeting drugs is to improve patient compliance and to ensure site specific drug delivery and long action duration. These are as follows:

1. Prodrugs:

    Inactive drug forms which are metabolised to form active drugs, thereby increasing usefulness of the drug .E.g. Levodopa is a prodrug which can cross the blood brain barrier and then gets converted to Dopamine , which in turn is utilised centrally to treat Parkinson's disease. Some prodrugs provide long duration of action like Procaine penicillin-G and Benzathine Penicillin-G

2. Computerised Miniature pumps:

    These are systems designed to release the drug at a constant rate. Sometimes a drug is released in pulses as in GnRH (Gonadotropin releasing hormone), or it may be released continuously as in Insulin Pumps, which are provided with Glucose sensor devices which release insulin depending on body's demand.

3. Ocuserts and Progestaserts:

    Ocuserts are drug reservoirs shaped into very thin elliptical devices. Drug is released via membrane through diffusion. E.g. Pilocarpine ocuserts find use in Glaucoma.

Progestaserts are intrauterine devices containing contraceptive agents placed in the uterus to release drugs at uniform rate.

4. Liposomes:

Phospholipids are sonicated as suspension in small vesicles. These drugs are released till degradation of vesicles. E.g. Amphotericin B in liposomal form is given as Intravenous infusion . It has benefits of being less toxic to the kidney , has better tolerability but is a little more expensive.

5. Monoclonal Antibodies becoming carriers for Drugs:

Monoclonal Antibodies (MAbs) are produced by single clones and are working against single antigenic determinants (*Epitope*). They are produced by *"Hybridoma Technique"*. Initially murine (derived from rodents) MAbs were developed, later modified to humanised MAbs by genetic techniques. These were now called *"Chimeric MAbs"*. Advantages of completely humanised MAbs are very low Antigenicity.

Naming of Monoclonal Antibodies:

- The name of all monoclonal antibodies end with "mab"
- Letter before "mab" indicates source. E.g. "o" for murine (omab), "xi" for chimeric, i.e. human mixed with rodents components (ximab), "zu" for humanised, i.e. more human, less rodent (zumab), "u" for fully human, (umab).

- Letter before above discussed ones stand for the purpose they serve, their use, E.g. "tu" for tumour (Rituximab), "vi" for virus (Palavizumab), "ci" for circulation (Abciximab). In case any such letters are not present, the purpose is simply of an immunomodulator.

<u>Dosage forms</u>

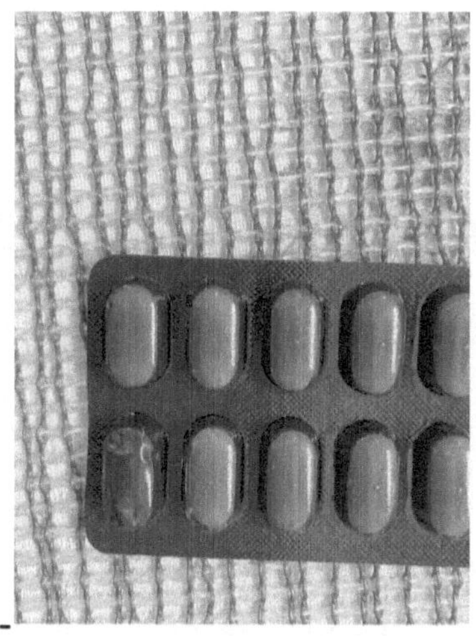

Analgesic Tablets (Solid dosage form)

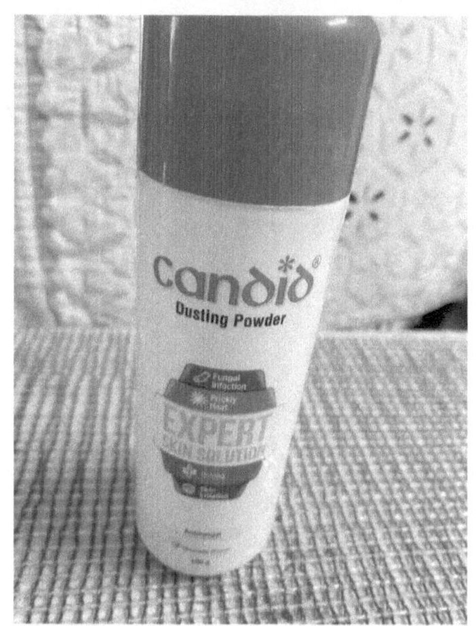

Dusting Powder (Solid dosage form)

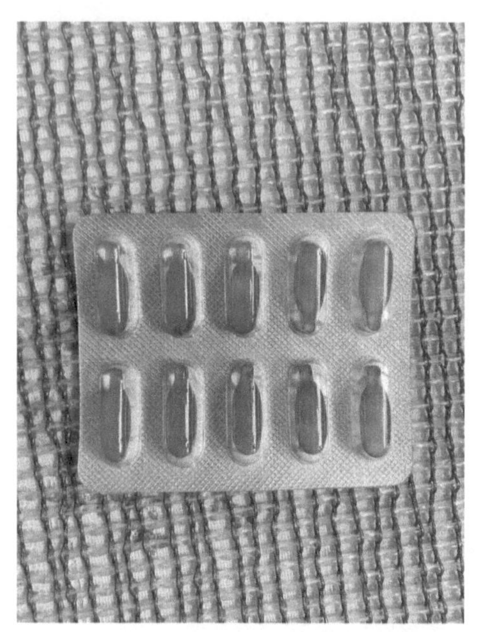

Soft Gel Capsules (Solid dosage forms)

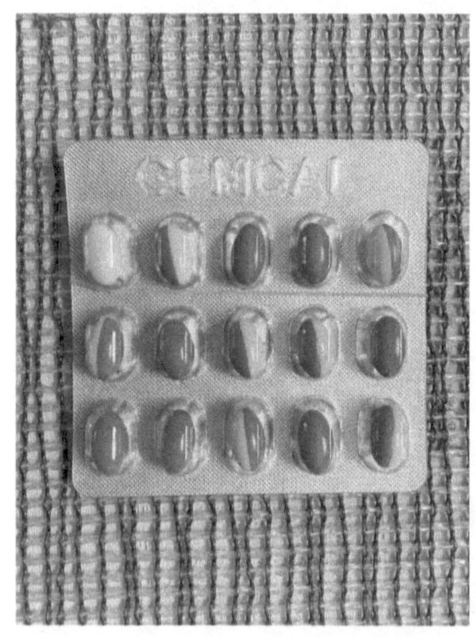

Soft Gelatin Capsules (Solid dosage forms)

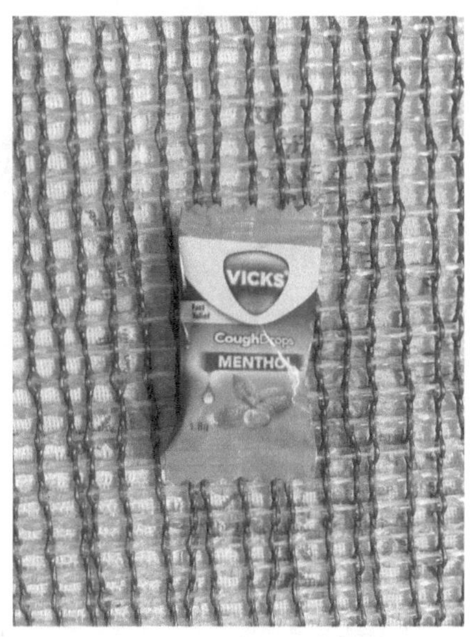

Vicks Lozenges (Solid dosage forms)

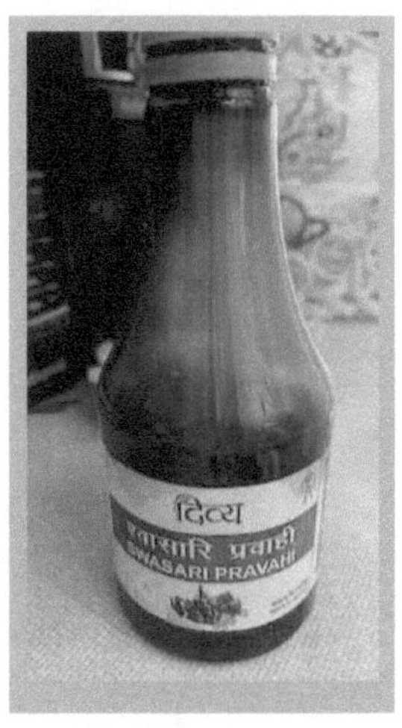

Cough Linctus (Liquid dosage form)

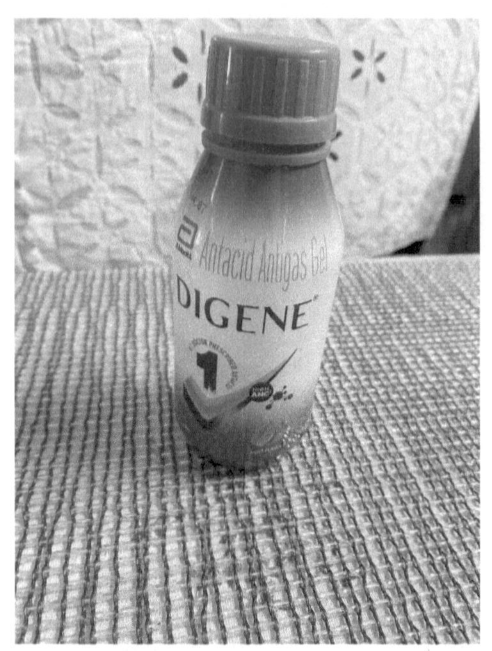

Antacid Gel (Liquid dosage form)

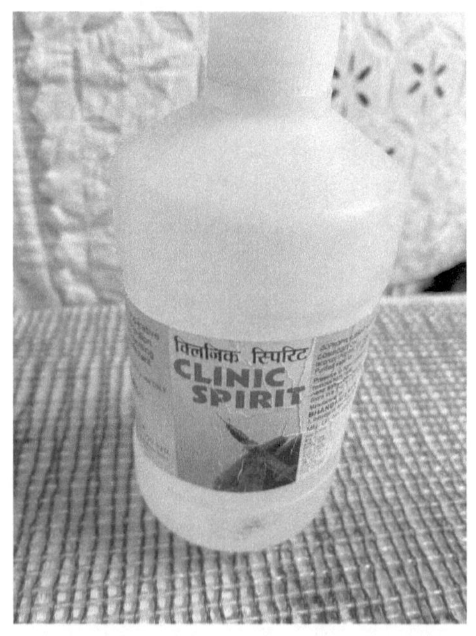

Spirit (Liquid dosage form)

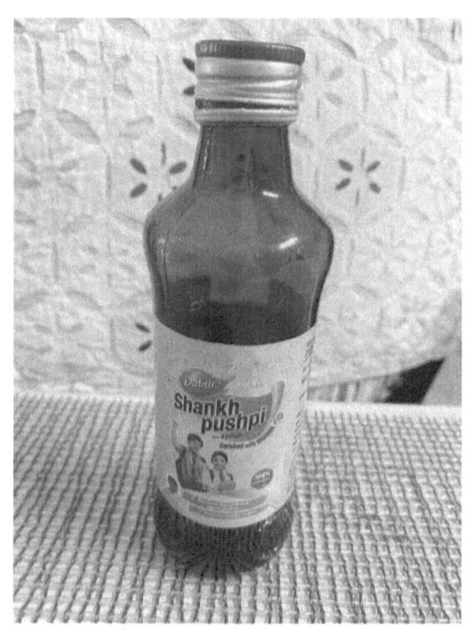

Syrup (Liquid dosage form)

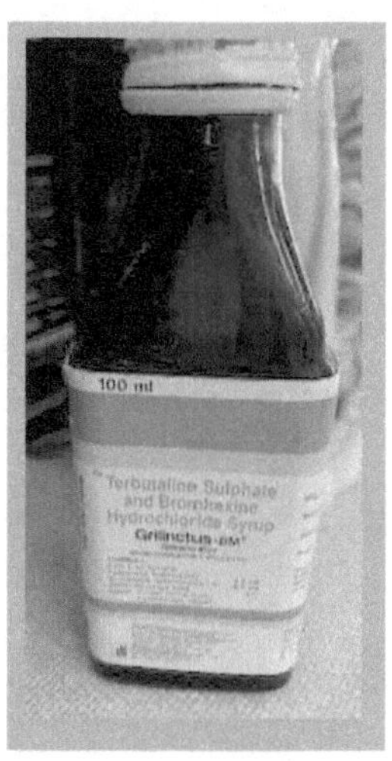

Cough Syrup (Liquid dosage form)

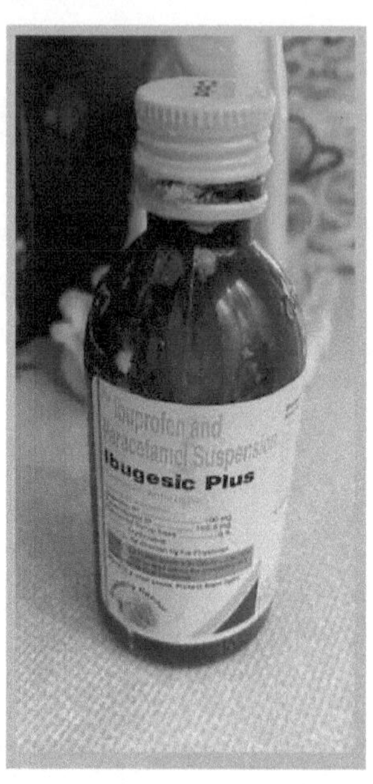

Analgesic Suspension (Liquid dosage form)

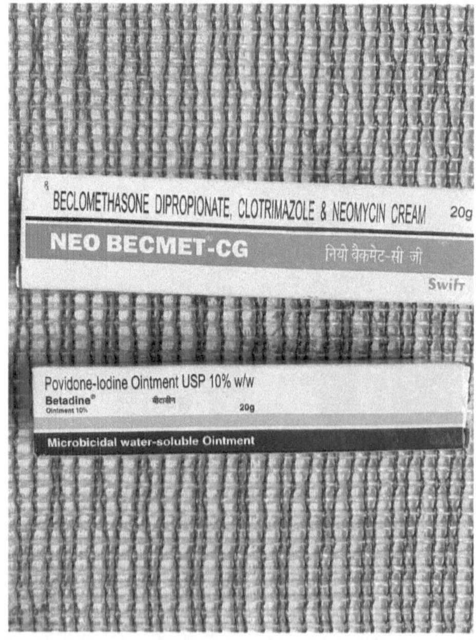

Antimicrobial Cream and Ointment (Semisolid dosage form)

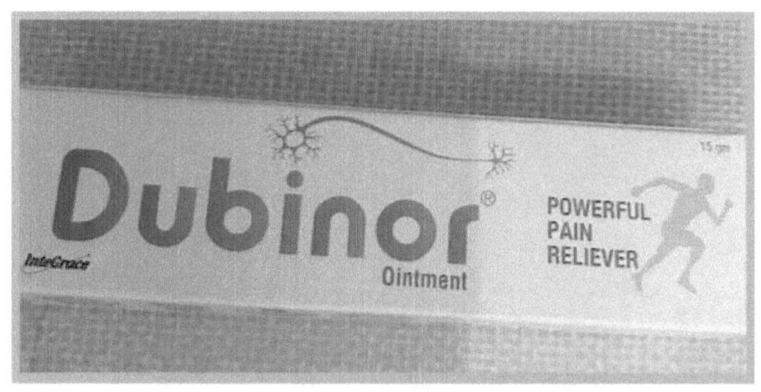

Ointment (Semi solid dosage form)

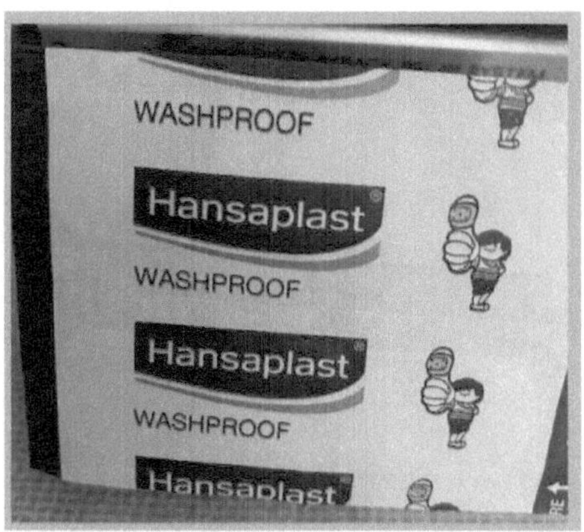

Band-aid (Semi solid dosage form)

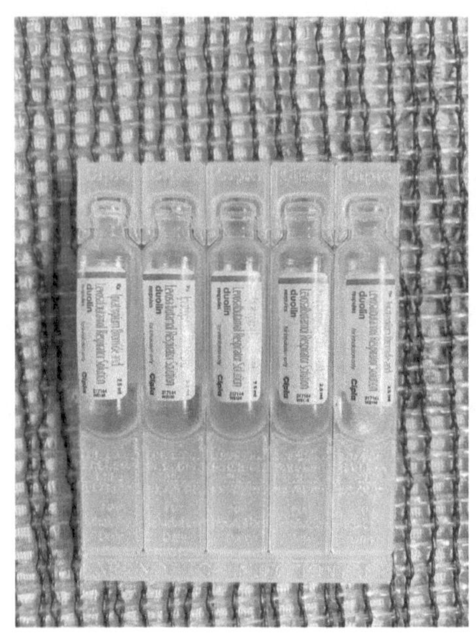

Respules (Inhalational suspension -Dosage form for nebuliser)

Drug Absorption

Definition:

Movement of drugs from the site of administration into the blood circulation is called Absorption.

Factors governing the process of Absorption:

1. Water Solubility- It is an important deciding factor about the rate of drug absorption.It is a good rule for all solid drugs to dissolve nicely before absorption occurs, but if the drug is not water soluble (Propranolol, Timolol, Griseofulvin), its rate of dissolution decides the pattern of its absorption. Generally water soluble drugs absorb faster than lipid soluble drugs.

2. Blood circulation of Absorption site- Increased blood circulation enhances the removal of drug from the site thereby hastening the process of absorption.

3. Route of drug Administration- Absorption varies with each route. It's quick via sublingual, intravenous route, while slow with oral route.

4. Area of absorbing surface- Absorption increases with increase in area of site of absorption.

5. Drug concentration- Concentrated drugs are absorbed faster than dilute drug solutions.

Characteristics of Absorption via different routes of drug administration.

★ Oral:

Particle size is an important determining factor as far as absorption rate is concerned. Smaller particles dissolve easily and are absorbed fast. Presence of food dilutes the drug and delays gastric emptying and slows down absorption. If complexes are formed in between drug and food chemicals, the absorption suffers.Highly ionised drugs are not absorbed orally e.g. neostigmine.

Some exceptions being that a fat rich diet enhances absorption of highly lipid soluble foods like griseofulvin (antifungal) and piperaquine (antimalarial). Gastric acid destroys some of the drugs like insulin, penicillin, hence they are not given orally. For the same reason, Enteric coated tablets of few drugs like Aspirin, diclofenac sodium, bisacodyl, diltiazem are much in vogue. And Sustained release tablets of Metformin, Praocainamide, Progesterone, etc are made to protect drugs from direct contact of gastric acid.

P-gp is an efflux transporter that restricts the absorption of drugs like digoxin, cyclosporin. Hence inducers (rifampicin, phenytoin) of P-gp further reduce absorption of these drugs, while inhibitors (verapamil, erythromycin) enhance their absorption. Other factors in this head include drug complex formation in lumen (chelating agents, tetracyclines, sucralfate), changes in gut motility(opioids, anticholinergics), gastric mucosa damaging drugs(methotrexate,NSAIDs)

★ Parenteral:

When drugs are given via Subcutaneous (s.c.) or Intramuscular (i.m.) routes, they get assimilated around capillaries, further lipid solubility matters, but in fact large lipid insoluble drugs too pass through capillaries via paracellular spaces. Still larger drugs are absorbed via lymphatics. So there is a good scope of many drugs to be absorbed parenterally which miss their chance via oral route. Parenteral routes are aiding in fast drug absorption, they have benefits of being consistent, stable. Though absorption from i.m. site is faster than s.c. site. E.g.Drugs like Insulin, opioids, heparin, adrenaline and some antiallergic medicines are given via s.c. route while antibiotics (benzathine penicillin, streptomycin), biologicals (vaccines, immunoglobulins), hormones (medroxyprogesterone, testosterone) are given i.m.

★ Topical:

If the drug is highly lipid soluble, a certain degree of systemic absorption too occurs , Though a few names to count on fingers are corticosteroids, Glyceryl trinitrate, nicotine, estradiol, etc. To enhance absorption, techniques like rubbing, occlusive dressing, etc can be used. Absorption via abraded surfaces is faster and can produce systemic toxicity. Physostigmine being a tertiary compound is used as eye drops in Glaucoma and it can penetrate the cornea. Topical surfaces of mouth, rectum, vagina also absorb lipid soluble drugs and their systemic effects are seen.

Bioavailability Of Drugs

Definition:

As per USFDA, "The rate at which and extent to which the active drug concentration is available at site of action is called as Bioavailability of a drug".

- Fraction of administered dose of drug that reaches systemic circulation without undergoing any alterations is known as Bioavailability of drugs.

- It can be determined by either measuring the area under the Concentration time curve or simply by drug excretion in urine.

- If a drug is injected by I.V. route, its bioavailability is 100%. When a drug is given by oral route, the bioavailability decreases as the drug may be incompletely absorbed or it may be subjected to first pass metabolism. Local drug binding after s.c. or i.m. injection also reduces drug bioavailability.

- Bioavailability is an absolute term, while Equivalence is a relative term. Latter refers to comparison of two brands of the same drug with set standards.

- Pharmaceutical factors (involves rate and extent of disintegration and dissolution of drugs) like size of particle, salt/crystal form, hydration water content, nature of excipients, adjuvants and degree of ionisation affect the bioavailability of drugs.

- Pharmacological factors like gastrointestinal motility (bioavailability increases with all the factors increasing gastric emptying like fasting, anxiety, lying on the right side, drugs like metoclopramide an decreases with decreasing factors like fatty diet, endogenous depression, hypothyroidism, drugs like atropine, etc), various gastrointestinal pathological states like coeliac disease, crohn's disease and gastroenteritis affect the bioavailability of drug in variegated pattern. Empty stomach generally favors gastrointestinal drug absorption, and certain drugs, especially antibiotics (rifampicin) decrease the rate and extent of drug absorption. First pass metabolism decreases net bioavailability of drugs. Drug - drug interactions exhibit unpredictable effects on drug absorption, pharmacogenetic states like presence or absence of atypical pseudocholinesterase also affects bioavailability of drugs and miscellaneous features like route of drug administration, surface area of absorption and circulation state combinedly affect the drug's bioavailability.

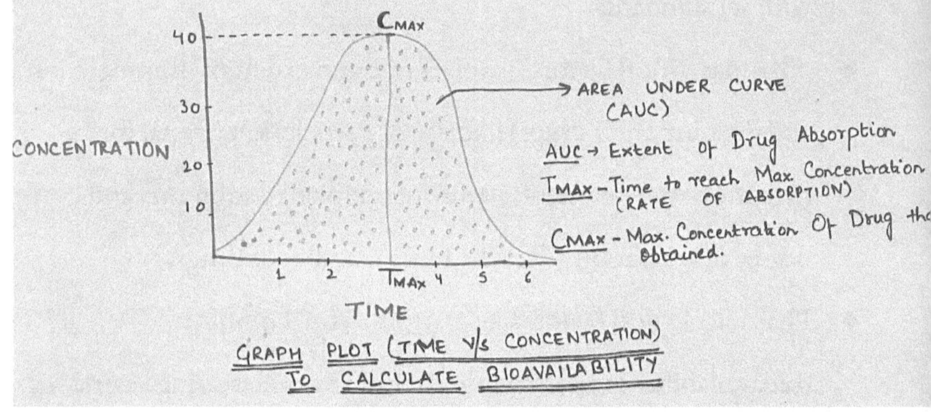

Fig 4. Bioavailability Graph

Different types of Equivalences are:

- Bioequivalence:

  When two drug preparations contain the same amount of drug , though they are from different manufacturing companies, and they exhibit the same levels of drug plasma concentrations achieved, then they are known as Bioequivalent (biologically equivalent) drugs/ drug preparations. E.g. Dilantin (Park Davis) and Eptoin (Boots) both are chemically Phenytoin but may or may not be Bioequivalent.

Less than 25% difference in bioavailability is insignificant and still if all other criteria met, drug

can be called Bioequivalent.

Importance: Drug regulatory authorities (DCGI in India and FDA in USA) always lay stress on

evidence of bioequivalence of drugs so that Generic drug can be conveniently changed to its

Branded drug with no changes in therapeutic or clinical drug effects. For drugs with steep

dose-response relation (phenytoin, warfarin) and drugs with narrow safety margin (theophylline,

cyclosporine) switching of brands should be avoided as this may result in either drug failure or

drug intoxication.

- Chemical Equivalence:

  When two or more dosage forms of the same drug contain the same drug amount as stated in pharmacopoeia, then they are Chemically equivalent.

- Therapeutic Equivalence:

  When two or more brand preparations of the same drug exhibit the same response inside the body, they are called therapeutically equivalent.

- Pharmaceutical Equivalence:

Along with the main ingredient, if additives, excipients, other agents (binders, flavours, colours) are also the same in two or more drug forms, then they are called pharmaceutically equivalent.

- Clinical Equivalence:

When one or more structurally different drugs produce the same clinical response as other related drugs, they are said to be clinically equivalent. E.g. Trifluoperazine (phenothiazine) and Haloperidol (butyrophenone) exhibit similar results for schizophrenia and are called clinically equivalent.

Drug Distribution

Once the absorption process is complete, the drug enters the systemic circulation and gets distributed.

There are many factors on which drug distribution depends like lipid solubility, ionisation at physiological pH, presence or absence of tissue specific receptors and plasma protein binding.

Apparent Volume of Distribution:

Definition: The volume of drug that would accommodate all the amount of drug in the body , if there had been the same concentration everywhere as in plasma.We can know its amount in multiples of that in unit volume in plasma.

Formula can be given as:

$$V=(\text{Dose administered i.v.}/\text{plasma concentration})$$

- Highly plasma protein bound drugs (warfarin, theophylline, chloroquine) stay strictly in the vascular compartment, and their volume of distribution is very less.

- Large amounts of extravascular drugs generally show a large volume of distribution. Drugs like digoxin, morphine having a large volume of distribution are deposited in tissues. For such drug toxicities, even hemodialysis is not useful.

- Diseases like Congestive heart failure, liver cirrhosis, uremia, etc, value of distribution volume is highly affected.

Plasma Protein Binding

Binding of drugs to the plasma proteins is referred to as Plasma Protein Binding (PPB). This binding is due to the drugs' physicochemical nature and is many times reversible in nature. Acidic drugs (Penicillins, Warfarin, Barbiturates, etc.) bind to plasma Albumin and basic drugs (Quinidine, Verapamil, lidocaine, etc.) bind to alpha-1 acid glycoprotein

From this we infer that:

- If a drug is highly plasma protein bound, it stays in the vascular compartment and exhibits small volumes of distribution.

- Plasma protein binding as Storage -
  After binding, bound and free form generally stay in equilibrium. If there is more excretion of free drug, bound drug dissociates and serves to act as free drug.

- Long action duration of bound drug-
  Once a drug is highly bound to plasma proteins, it becomes long acting. The bound fraction of drug is not available for action or metabolism or excretion. If in case toxicity of these drugs ensues, it's not helped by haemodialysis, other treatment techniques are needed.

- Drug displacement reactions-

One drug can bind to many sites, many drugs can bind to one site. The drugs with higher affinity generally displace those with lower affinity (and in turn increase the free form of latter drug).

- Disease states:

In different diseases, PPB varies as per increase and decrease in binding proteins. In hypoalbuminemia, high concentrations of free drugs are present (acidic drug), In uremia, pethidine binding is lowered. In pregnancy and acute inflammation, alpha-1 acid glycoprotein is raised, so basic drug binding is enhanced.

Redistribution

Definition:

Redistribution is defined as the process of distribution which causes significant change in drug plasma concentration so that it is enough to terminate the drug's action.

- It is a feature of highly lipid soluble drugs
- This type of redistribution is after the first phase of distribution, it is the second phase. Initially the drug is distributed to highly vascular organs like the brain, heart, liver, kidney. Later it moves out of these organs due to high degree of blood flow, and gets

distributed peripherally. Actin of drug at the main site fades away or gets terminated.

- Example is of thiopentone sodium, a short acting barbiturate , it gets quickly redistributed and its action terminates.

- One quick trick to elongate action duration of drug undergoing redistribution is to give the drug frequently many times or continuously for long durations. This can make the drug longer acting.

Drug distribution in Brain (CSF) , Placenta and Tissues

- In Brain:

The Blood Brain Barrier is present in the brain, it is composed of layers of capillary endothelial cells (having tight junctions) and neural tissue. The blood-CSF barrier lies in the choroid plexus. Both the barriers allow entry of lipid soluble drugs/substances. BBB is deficient at CTZ in medulla oblongata.

Here one can find primary and secondary active carriers like P-gp and OATP too which expel out harmful compounds and are protective in nature.

In meningeal bacterial infections and other inflammatory states, permeability increases manifold so as to allow sometimes entry of lipid insoluble compounds too.

Enzymatic Blood Brain Barrier is composed of specific enzymes like cholinesterase, MAO, etc and restrict entry of their respective substrates like Acetylcholine , 5-HT, etc.

- In Placenta:

Lipid soluble drugs easily pass through the placenta. P-gp and transporters like BCRP and MRP3 limit harmful substances by efflux mechanism. Drug metabolism also occurs in Placenta. Though it is an incomplete barrier and hence mothers are advised to not take any drug during pregnancy and also after child birth.

- In Tissues:

Once lipid soluble drugs enter tissues they may accumulate through process of active transport or may especially bind to tissue parts like digoxin accumulates in heart, kidney and muscles; tetracyclines accumulates and damages teeth and bones; chloroquine binds to nucleoproteins in the eye.

Drugs have a large volume of distribution in the tissues and long action duration. Sometimes their high concentration turns out to be very dangerous and ensues local toxicity (examples above).

Drug Biotransformation /Drug Metabolism

Definition:

All reactions leading to changes in drugs chemically in the body refer to the drug biotransformation. The result is that lipid soluble compound changes to water soluble and it can be further easily excreted.

Primarily drug metabolism occurs in the liver. Other sites are Kidney, lungs, intestine, etc.

Consequences of Biotransformation may be:

1. To Inactivate drug:

   Active drugs and their metabolites (lidocaine, paracetamol, ibuprofen, etc.) are made inactive and finally excreted.

2. Formation of Active drug metabolite:

   Many active drugs are converted to Active metabolites (Digitoxin to digoxin, Codeine to Morphine, Spironolactone to Canrenone, etc). The combined effect of Parent drug and active metabolite defines the complete final response.

3. To activate inactive drug:

   Some drugs are initially inactive and require a conversion to active drugs or metabolites to perform action. Such inactive drugs are known as *Prodrugs*

Advantages of Prodrugs:

- More stable

- Less side effects

- Better bioavailability

- Desirable features in their pharmacokinetics.

Examples include-

Levodopa to Dopamine, Prednisone to Prednisolone, Proguanil to Cycloguanil, Becampicillin to Ampicillin, etc.

Types Of Biotransformation Reactions

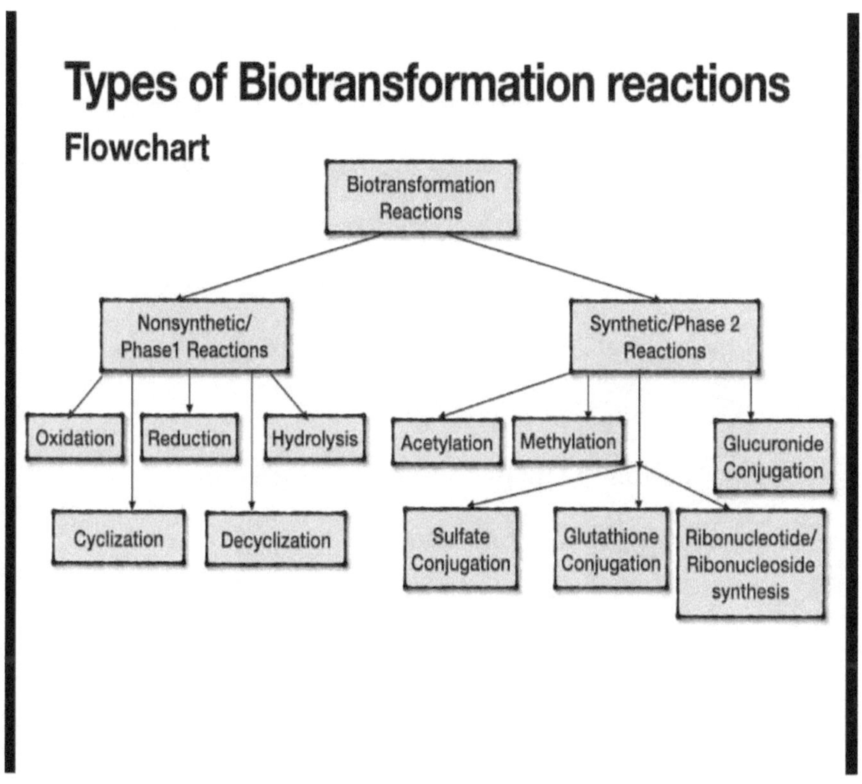

(a) Non synthetic/Phase 1 Reactions:

A functional group is attached (-OH, -COOH, -NH2), hence the reaction is also known as Functionalization reaction, metabolite generated may be active or inactive.

Major Non Synthetic reactions are as follows:

- Oxidation- In this oxygen is added, mainly reaction is carried out with the help of monooxygenases in the liver.E.g. Barbiturates, paracetamol, steroids, etc.

- Reduction-its the opposite of oxidation, Cytochrome-P450 enzymes act reverse.E.g. Chloramphenicol, Halothane, Warfarin, etc.

- Hydrolysis-In this water molecule is taken up to cleave the drug

Ester + H2O------------Acid+Alcohol

Esterases

Amidases and Peptidases perform the same action on Amines and Peptides. Hydrolysis occurs mainly in Liver, intestine, etc. E.g. Aspirin, Procaine, lidocaine, Pethidine, etc.

- Cyclization- A ring structure is formed from a linear compound. E.g. Cycloguanil from proguanil.

- Decyclization- This is opposite of above, the linear compound is obtained back from the ring structure.E.g. Phenytoin.

(b) Synthetic/ Phase 2 Reactions:

The drug conjugates with an endogenous compound, resulting in a metabolite that is mostly inactive and easily excreted in urine or bile. These reactions are also termed as Conjugation reactions. Exceptions being Glucuronide conjugate of morphine and sulfate conjugate of minoxidil which are active compounds. These reactions are speedy in nature and require energy.

If the drug already consists of a functional group, its direct conjugation will occur, else the drug goes through phase 1 reaction followed by phase 2 reaction.

Major Synthetic Reactions are as follows:

- Glucuronide Conjugation

  This is the most important synthetic reaction. UDP Glucuronosyl Transferases (UGTs) are utilised to make the process happen. E.g. Paracetamol, Aspirin, Morphine, etc. Along with these endogenous substances like thyroxine, bilirubin, etc can also be conjugated.

  The Resulting compound is heavy, it is easily excreted in bile. If these compounds are acted upon by gut bacteria, the drug is dissociated and reabsorbed, and the vicious cycle continues. This is termed as *Enterohepatic Cycling,* which makes the drug long acting. E.g. OCPs.

- Acetylation:

  Acetyl coenzyme-A conjugates drugs possessing Amino or Hydrazine residues, like Isoniazid, PAS, Dapsone, Hydralazine, etc. Enzyme involved is N-Acetyl Transferases (NATs). Genetic polymorphism is exhibited, the drug may be Slow or fast Acetylator.

- Glutathione conjugation:

  This is a minor yet important metabolic pathway. Glutathione S Transferase (GST) carries out this reaction. During paracetamol poisoning, a large volume of highly dangerous and reactive intermediate species of radicals like epoxide or quinone are formed, due to this , there occurs shortage of Glutathione, all this toxic environment damages vital organs like liver, kidney, etc. GST works to inactivate the highly toxic and reactive intermediate radicals.

- Miscellaneous:

These include many minor yet important pathways like Methylation, Sulfate conjugation, Glycine conjugation, Ribonucleotide or ribonucleoside synthesis.

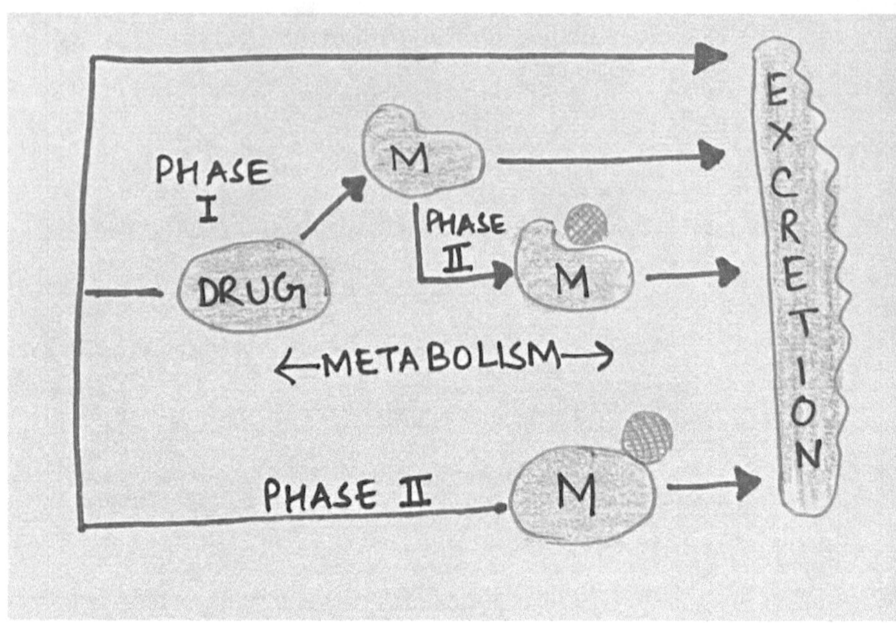

Fig 5. Phase 1 and Phase 2 metabolism of Drug In sequence

(M=Metabolite)

Drug Metabolising Enzymes

Almost all drugs are acted upon by drug metabolising Enzymes which can be broadly divided in two types:

1. Microsomal enzymes:

   They are found mainly in Liver, kidney, lungs, intestine, etc. They are specifically located on the Smooth Endoplasmic reticulum. E.g. Monooxygenases, cytochrome P450, etc.They can be induced as well as inhibited. Many reactions like oxidation, hydrolysis, reduction are catalysed by these enzymes and Glucuronide conjugation too!

2. Non Microsomal Enzymes:

   They are found in mitochondria and cytoplasm in cells of the liver , plasma, various tissues, etc. E.g. esterases, amidases, most conjugases, etc. Many reactions are catalysed by these enzymes like oxidations, reduction, almost all conjugations except Glucuronide Conjugation. These enzymes exhibit Genetic Polymorphism (N-acetyl transferase)

Cytochrome P-450 (CYP) Isoenzymes

- More than 100 different types of CYP isoenzymes have been discovered along with their respective substrates. In humans few members of mainly 3 families (CYP 1,2,3) carry out almost all metabolic reactions. Most important ones are:

    - CYP3A4/5- More than 50% of drugs are their substrates.

    - CYP2D6- Almost 20% drugs are their substrates. Due to Inhibition of CYP2D6 by quinidine , the conversion of codeine to morphine does not occur, hence no analgesia.

    - CYP2C8/9- More than 15 drugs (phenytoin, carbamazepine) are their substrates.

    - CYP2C19- More than 12 drugs (Omeprazole, diazepam) are their substrates.

    - CYP1A1/2- Only few drugs (theophylline, caffeine, paracetamol) are their substrates, they are involved in procarcinogen activation.

    - CYP2E1- It is utilised in oxidation of alcohol, halothane, formation of toxic metabolite in paracetamol poisoning.

- As far as Nomenclature of CYP Isoenzymes is concerned, they are classified in variety of families denoted by a number 1,2,3, 4, etc. the subfamilies are denoted by sequence of amino acid and c-DNA cloning studies and written as capital letter A,B,C,D, etc. One more number is written thereafter which denotes specific isoenzymes. E.g. in CYP2D6, the family is 2, subfamily s D, gene number is 6. Most common three subfamilies CYP3A, CYP2D, CYP2C and CYP2E are of importance to us; these exhibit genetic polymorphism.

- A drug can inhibit or induce these isoenzymes.
- Enzyme Inhibition:

In this, the drug inhibits the drug metabolising Isoenzyme, thereby increasing the substrate concentration and sometimes this also predisposes to toxicity of the object drug.

This process occurs within hours, it's a speedy reaction.

Hepatic blood flow limits metabolism of few drugs which are highly extracted by the liver (Lidocaine, morphine, verapamil).

Sometimes a drug may inhibit its own metabolism (Verapamil) .

- Enzyme Induction:

When enzyme protein synthesis is increased especially P-450 and UGTs, this is termed as Enzyme Induction.

Induction involves enzymes found in all organs along with mainly the liver, and it takes time, around 5 days to 2 weeks to exhibit maximum effect. Once the agent is stopped, the enzymes regain their normal form and shape.

As a result, the substrate drug concentration and effect decreases (failure of contraception when OCP is given along with rifampicin)

Sometimes a drug is activated by metabolism, then an overall enhanced effect is observed.

Sometimes Tolerance develops in case the drug induces self metabolism , i.e. AutoInduction (Nevirapine, Carbamazepine)

If inducer is applied intermittently, it may lead to disturbed and erratic results.

Along with normal induction reactions, some endogenous substances like bilirubin, etc may too get induced.

Enzyme Induction increases porphyrin synthesis by depressing delta-aminolevulinic acid synthetase and in turn leads to development of acute intermittent porphyria.

Enzyme induction can be used for benefit purposes therapeutically and clinically:

- In case of poisonings, it helps by quick metabolism of the poison.

- In case of Cushing Syndrome, Phenytoin may enhance metabolism of steroids found in excess.

- In case of Congenital Nonhemolytic kernicterus in the newborn , there is lacking Glucuronidation of bilirubin, hence phenytoin helps by clearing away bilirubin/jaundice.

- It is of great help in liver diseases.

First Pass Metabolism/ Pre Systemic Metabolism

As the drug goes through the different sites of absorption, finally to enter the blood circulation, it gets metabolised on its way upto a certain extent, this is known as First Pass Effect/ First Pass metabolism/ Pre Systemic Metabolism. This is bound to occur with Oral drugs. Certain routes of drug administration (Sublingual, parenteral) almost completely bypasses this effect. First Pass Metabolism is an important factor contributing to the drug bioavailability.

If a drug has high first pass metabolism, keep the oral dose higher as compared to other routes. Apply the same high oral dose in case of liver diseases too.

Non Enzymatic Biotransformation (Hofmann Elimination)

Definition:

Some drugs are metabolised spontaneously in plasma through the Molecular rearrangement process . In this, there is no involvement of any enzyme action. Such non enzymatic biotransformation of drugs is called *Hofmann Elimination.* E.g. Atracurium (Skeletal Muscle Relaxant)

Factors Affecting Drug Metabolism

There are many factors affecting drug metabolism. The most important ones are :

1. Age and Sex:

   Extremes of ages show strikingly different patterns of metabolism, in small children, low activity of enzyme Glucuronyl transferase is found which makes them prone to conditions like "Grey baby syndrome" due to the drug Chloramphenicol. Elderly people, > 60 years of age have decreased flow of blood to the liver. This slows down the metabolism of drugs like pethidine and propranolol and precipitate their toxicity.

   As far as sex differences are concerned, it holds very little significance in human beings, Though its of some importance as stated by animal studies (Due to effect of hexobarbital, male rats possessing high enzyme activity than females sleep for shorter time span)

2. Race and Species:

   As far as race is concerned, it holds some importance for humans like Chinese people who possess high alcohol dehydrogenase activity while low aldehyde dehydrogenase activity, hence after alcohol consumption , they exhibit high aldehyde blood plasma concentration. Species dependent metabolism variations are exhibited by Rabbits as they have high *Atropine esterase* activity in liver and plasma as compared to humans so they metabolise Atropine faster.

3. Nutrition and Diet:

Rich protein diet favours metabolic rate as it supplies glycine and cysteine essential to form conjugated drug metabolites. While a carbohydrate rich diet decreases metabolic rate.

4. Genetic differences:

It plays important role in drug metabolism as shown by the table:

Inherited defect	Object Drug	Clinical result
Atypical pseudocholinest erase	Succinylcholine (Neuromuscula r blocker)	Prolonged Apnoea
Slow Acetylator---- Fast Acetylators-----	Isoniazid (Antitubercular drug)	Neuropathy condition Hepatotoxicity
CYP2D6 Defective expression	Codeine (opioid)	Decreased level of Analgesia

Table 3. Examples of Genetic variations amongst people

5. Disease state and Drug Interactions:

    Diseases like hepatitis, liver cirrhosis, hepatocellular cancer and
    heavy metal poisoning slows down drug metabolism, while in
    states of hyperthyroidism, metabolism of drugs like digoxin is
    enhanced. Drug-drug interactions are shown by *Enzyme
    Inhibition* and *Enzyme Induction* processes.

DRUG METABOLISM ROLE IN DRUG DEVELOPMENT

Efficacy and Safety both are important elements for Drug Development.
When there is profound knowledge of drug metabolising enzymes for the
Novel drug candidate, then consequently a lot of knowledge will be gained
regarding future possible drug drug interaction and susceptibility to
Genetic Polymorphism.

Once the drug effectively undergoes the preclinical testing in animal
models, then it should be tested in human clinical study models.
Similarly, studies and analysis can be done with transporters and phase 2
enzymes which further clarifies the drug metabolism in future.

Receptor based studies help to find out parameters like drug binding
affinity, activation/depression and bioavailability, clearance etc.

Computer based computations (in silico) strongly predict drug
metabolism features for novel candidates. Enzyme and receptor structure
will be known.

Extent of drug toxicity and organ damage - when well known in preclinical studies, can guide very well in drug development, especially in development of lead compounds.

"Metabolomics" is used along with HTS to identify toxicity biomarkers. Metabolomics can be defined as systematic identification and quantification of all metabolites in an organism or sample.

Comparative analysis of a lot of chemicals in biological fluids like urine, etc can be easily done with association of techniques like liquid chromatography, mass spectrometry, etc.

Filtering and scanning the needful pathological treatments and drug toxicities on thousands of animals can be judged for their relevance and aptness easily and accurately. This can in turn give way to judge and analyse efficacy and toxicity of a drug in patients receiving pharmacotherapy. Consequently, drug responders and non responders are easily identified.

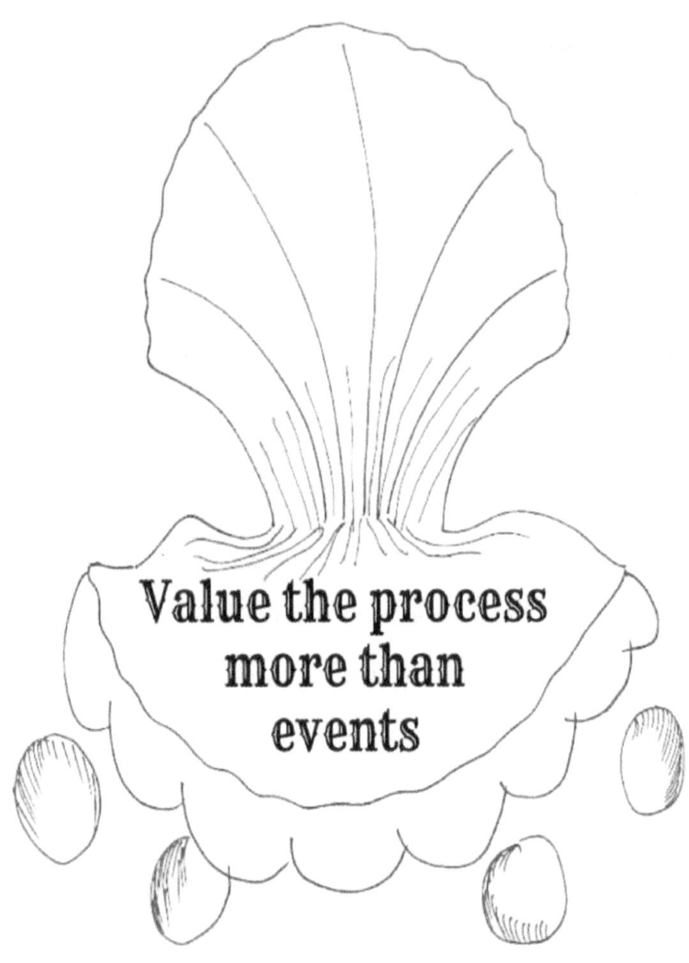

Value the process
more than
events

Chapter 3

Pharmacokinetics at a Glance-2

KEY FEATURES

- *Routes Of Drug Elimination*
- *Kinetics of Elimination*
- *Clearance*
- *Plasma Half Life*
- *Drug Dosing*
- *Therapeutic drug Monitoring*

Definition:

Expulsion of drugs after being absorbed and biotransformed out of the body is called Drug Excretion or Elimination of Drugs.

Routes of Drug Elimination

There are many routes via which the drug can be eliminated out of the body. The main being renal route which is discussed in utter detail . Along with this, let us enlist some more of the routes found in the body for drug elimination:

1. Renal route of Drug excretion:

This is the major route of drug excretion via urine. Three key processes add up to decide the final fate of a drug via kidney.

Net renal Excretion= (Glomerular Filtration+Tubular Secretion)-Tubular Reabsorption

- Glomerular Filtration:

  All types of drugs (Lipid/Water Soluble) entering the Glomeruli get filtered as pores in Glomerular capillaries are large. In a way, PPB and Renal vascular flow finally determine the Glomerular filtration.Normal g.f.r (Glomerular Filtration Rate) = 120ml/min

- Tubular secretion:

  There are two separate transporter systems , namely OAT and OCT, which operate in proximal kidney tubules responsible for active transfer of Organic acids and bases respectively. This is the Tubular Secretion of Drugs. Along with these efflux transporters like P-gp and MRP2 also operate.

  This process helps in more degradation of protein bound drugs which can be further secreted and eliminated. Hence PPB is no obstacle for this process, rather in a way it helps.

Organic Acid transport (OATP) works great for drugs like salicylates, methotrexate, penicillin, etc. Organic Base Transport (OCT) works for drugs like furosemide, thiazides, cimetidine, etc.

Generally both above discussed transporters work in two directional patterns, but secretion of drugs and metabolites in the tubular lumen is much prioritized and preferred system of transport. Uric Acid being an endogenous compound is mostly reabsorbed.

Drug displacement reactions are a common feature at sites shared for more than one drug. Drugs compete with each other for the secretion process. E.g. Probenecid having great affinity for OATP , it has been seen to block active transport of both penicillin and uric acid. But penicillin is mostly secreted, its excretion decreases, and uric acid is mostly reabsorbed, hence its secretion (excretion) increases.

- Tubular Reabsorption:

The process involves Passive Diffusion. Drug Ionisation and lipid solubility are determining factors. The principle is defined by:

- Highly ionised drugs like aminoglycosides have their rate of excretion almost equal to g.f.r.

- Acidic urine favours ionisation and excretion of weak bases.

- Alkaline urine favours ionisation and excretion of weak acids.

These points explain the treatment of poisoning of few drugs, like urine is acidified for poisoning of weak bases (morphine, codeine, amphetamine) and urine is made alkaline for poisoning of weak acids (barbiturates).

NOTE- These tubular mechanisms are not functional at birth, hence in the newborn, many drugs are long acting like penicillin. Renal function also deteriorates after 50 years of age, hence renal clearance is low in elderly.

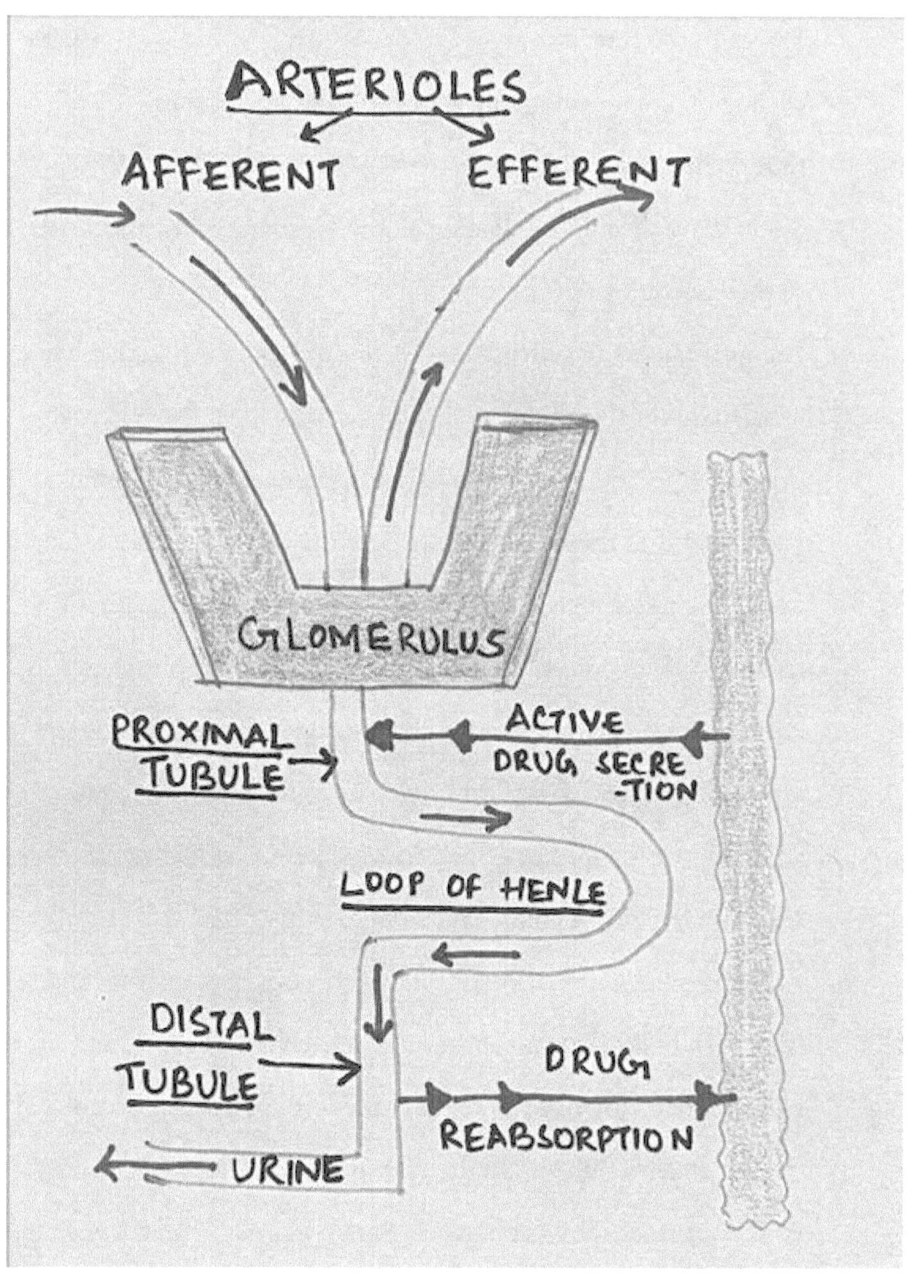

Fig 6. Renal excretion processes illustration

2. Faeces:In this, maximum drug is derived from bile. Enterohepatic cycling makes the drug long acting. E.g. Erythromycin, tetracycline, ampicillin, OCPs, etc.

3. Sweat and Saliva: Drugs like Lithium, KI, rifampicin are secreted in these secretions profusely.

4. Lungs (Exhaled air): Drugs like Alcohol, General Anaesthetics are exhaled out of the lung alveoli, This process depends on Partial pressure of blood. Lungs also help to eliminate harmful foreign particles out of the blood.

5. Milk: It is an important medium of drug transfer to the infant feeding on breast milk. The mechanism is quite simple. Drugs enter milk via Passive diffusion, Basic drugs accumulate more in low milk pH, hence very less drug reaches the infant, still it is advisable for the mothers not to take irrelevant medication for the sake of safety of the child.

6. Enterohepatic Circulation or Biliary excretion: Some drugs and drug metabolites (glucuronides) are delivered to the intestine after being secreted in bile , where these are deconjugated or hydrolysed (by gut enzymes) then they are reabsorbed back and the vicious cycle continues. This is known as *Enterohepatic Circulation.* This process serves as a small drug reservoir and helps to extend drug duration of action.E.g. thyroxine, morphine, ethinyl estradiol.

NOTE- In case of morphine poisoning, gastric lavage is indicated to avoid enterohepatic circulation and to prevent further damage.

Kinetics of Elimination

Definition:

Drug elimination defines the combined effect of both metabolic biotransformation (inactivation) of drug along with final excretion.

Importance:

1. Rational drug therapy is instituted by knowing the proper kinetics of Elimination.

2. Individual doses can be adopted and worked upon.

Clearance

Definition:

It is the volume of plasma from which a drug is completely removed in unit time. It can be calculated as follows:

$$\textbf{CL=Rate of Elimination /C}$$

Here C is the plasma concentration.

There are mainly two orders of kinetics:

1. First Order Kinetics:

In this, a constant *fraction* of drug present in the body is eliminated in unit time. Many of the drugs follow this order of kinetics (especially initially, later may saturate and shift to zero order)

- Elimination rate is directly proportional to the drug concentration
- CL remain constant
- t1/2 remains constant (as V and CL do not change)

2. Zero Order Kinetics:

In this, a constant *amount* of drugs is eliminated in unit time. E.g. ethyl alcohol.

- Rate of Elimination stays constant
- CL is indirectly proportional to the drug concentration.
- t1/2 is directly proportional to the dose of drug (as CL decreases with increase in dose)

This type of Elimination can be referred to as Capacity Limited Elimination or sometimes *Michaelis Menten elimination* (a kind of mixed order kinetics and dose dependent in nature, in which small doses are treated upon with first order kinetics but this changes to zero order at higher doses when metabolising enzymes or elimination procedure are saturated).

Some drugs show a shift from first Order to Zero order as and when their elimination process saturates . Sometimes drug elimination becomes blood flow dependent when the elimination ability of organs like liver, kidney etc. is much more than the amount of drug entering via blood circulation. Then these drugs are completely cleared off or excreted in a single passage through that organ.

Plasma Half Life

Definition:

Time taken for a drug to reduce its plasma concentration to half of the original value is termed as Plasma Half Life of the drug. When plotted as a plasma concentration-time graph, two major phases are observed:

1. Alpha phase- It is the initial rapidly declining phase, occurs due to drug distribution

2. Beta phase- It is the later slow declining phase, occurs due to drug elimination

Hence we can determine two half lives from the graph, but the major is elimination half life of the drug. The various steps of calculation of t1/2 (plasma half life) are as follows:

$$t1/2 = \ln2/k \qquad\qquad ....1.$$

Here, ln2=natural log of 2 (0.693)

k=elimination rate constant

$$k=CL/V \qquad \dots\dots\dots\dots 2.$$

Putting the appropriate values:

$$t1/2=0.693 * (V/CL) \qquad \dots\dots\dots\dots 3.$$

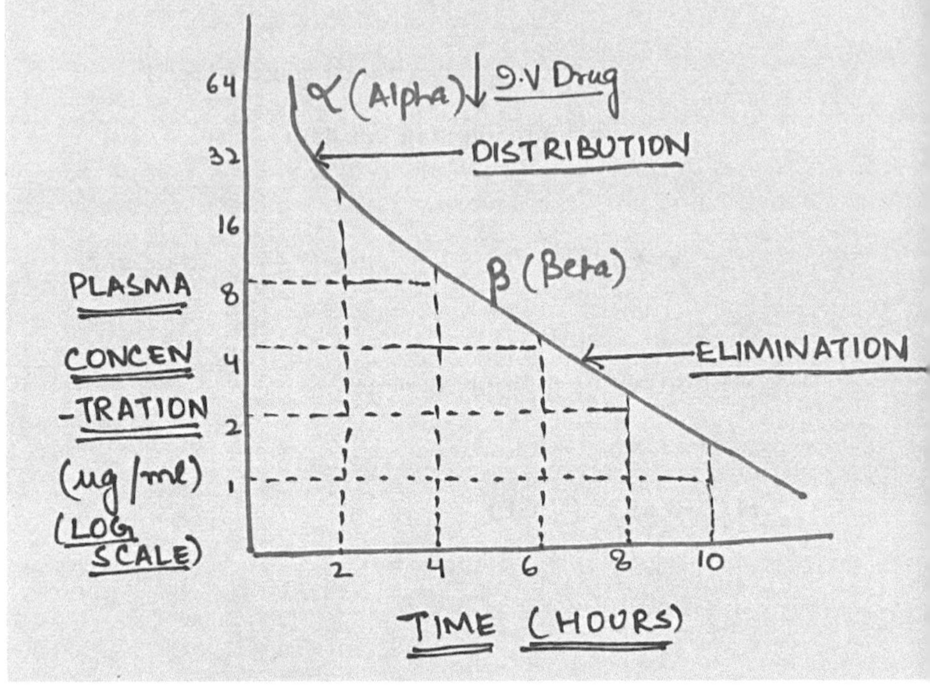

Fig 7. Plasma concentration V/S Time curve log graph of elimination of

drug via First order kinetics

(Shown are alpha and Beta components of plasma half life)

We infer that:

- Half life of a drug is dependent upon mainly two parameters, the Volume of drug distribution and Clearance of drug.

- After 1st half life--------50% drug is eliminated

  After 2nd half life-------75% drug is eliminated

  After 3rd half life-------87.5% drug is eliminated

After 4th half life--------93.75% drug is eliminated

Complete drug elimination occurs in 4-5 half lives.

- Examples of half lives of drugs, t1/2 of digoxin is 40 hours, t1/2 of digitoxin is 7 days, and t1/2 of Aspirin is 4 hours

Target Dose Strategy/ Concept of dual dosing

Plateau Principle:

On repeated drug administration, the drug accumulates in the body, till a steady state plasma concentration is achieved. On constantly giving the drug, it attains high peak concentration till 4-5 half lives. This process saturates when the amount of drug administered balances the rate of drug elimination.

Then the plasma concentration reaches a steady state level, it plateaus, hence the phenomenon is called the "*Plateau Principle*". This is generally reached in 4-5 half lives of the drug.

At steady state, the amplitude of drug plasma concentration fluctuates, and the difference between maximum and minimum heights is less if small doses are given repeatedly. Depending upon dosing frequency and acceptable levels of fluctuations, dose intervals are determined.

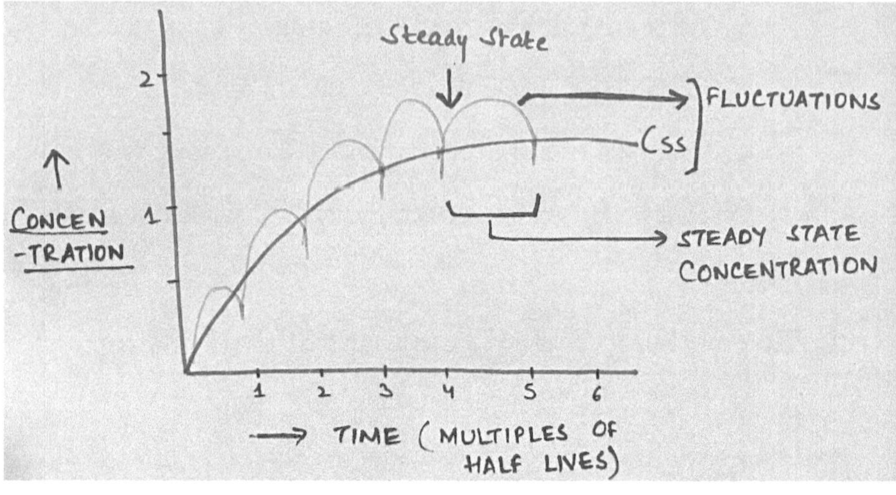

Fig 8. Steady state plasma concentration attained / Plateau principle

Target Dose Strategy/ Concept of dual dosing:

- This strategy is applied to drugs with low safety margin like antiepileptics, antiarrhythmics, antidepressants etc.

- Drugs with short t1/2 are given at set intervals.

- For Drugs with long t1/2 the strategy is to first administer a single loading dose and later on followed by maintenance doses.

- *Loading Dose:*

  It is either a single of few rapidly given doses to achieve target concentration rapidly . Its value is determined by only V (volume of drug distribution).

- *Maintenance Dose:*

This is a repeated dose administered at regular time intervals, once the target level is achieved, with an aim to maintain the drug level and balance its elimination.. This is determined by CL (or t1/2) of the drug.

- Benefits :

This strategy aims to achieve quick therapeutic responses of drugs and is safe too. E.g. Chloroquine, sulfonamides, digoxin, etc.

Drug Dosages and Dosing schedules

Following types of drug dosages are of importance:

1. Fixed Dose: In this type, desired therapeutic effects are achieved easily before toxic dose level is reached, E.g. Analgesics and Oral contraceptives

2. Variable dose: If this dose is given with crude adjustments, then fine adjustments make difficult to measure endpoint (depression, anxiety) , or may slowly alter as in thyrotoxicosis, or vary because of pathophysiological factors (analgesics, etc.), adrenocortical pharmacotherapy.

If the dose is given with fine adjustments, Vital functions changing fast under influence of dose alterations can be easily tracked provided the end point is known. E.g. Adrenocortical replacement therapy is covered here.

3. Maximum tolerated dose (MTD): Due to many undesirable effects, ideal therapeutic response is not achieved, the dose is increased till max unwanted effects start to fade away, E.g. Anticancer drugs, antimicrobial drugs.

4. Minimum tolerated dose: This is applied to long term adrenocortical steroid therapy in the state of immunological inflammations as in asthma and rheumatoid arthritis. In this case, the dose providing therapeutic effects is large enough so that its side effects are unavoidable . Safety comes first and hence incomplete results of therapy are obtained.

Now let us know the Different Dosing Schedules:

1. Drugs with a very short half life: drugs are given as constant I.V. infusion to keep up a steady level. (adrenaline-1 to 2 mins, dopamine-5 mins)

2. Drugs with short t1/2: If t1/2 is from 30 min to 2 hours, then there are problems, so if safety margin is high and drug obeys first order kinetics, it is administered every 6-8 hours (paracetamol-2 hours, cephalexin<1 hour)

3. Drugs with t1/2 around 4-12 hours: these are given at every half life interval

4. Drugs with medium t1/2: If t1/2 is around 12-24 hours, the drugs are administered at every 12 hour interval.

5. Drugs with longer t1/2: these drugs have high Vd (diazepam-40hrs;50-70lts , digoxin-40 rs;640 lts, chloroquine-40 hrs;130 lts), they accumulate in tissues, so approach varies as per demand. In no emergency, slow i.v. Infusion would work, in case of emergency, an initial priming or loading dose is given to achieve steady state plasma concentration, followed by a maintenance dose to maintain steady state achieved.

Therapeutic Drug monitoring (TDM)

Definition:

A process by which the drug dose is adjusted according to its concentration in the plasma is known as Therapeutic drug monitoring.

Important features:

- Applied to drugs having correlation in drug plasma level and response or state of poisoning.

- It's good for people exhibiting wide differences (inter and intra-individual) in pharmacokinetic (ADME) parameters

- It is done for drugs having low safety margin like theophylline, anticonvulsants, antiarrhythmics, antidepressants , Lithium, etc.

- It is applied to drugs whose responses are difficult to measure accurately like it is not applied for antihypertensives (BP measurement) , Anticoagulants, antidiabetics, etc. It is not applied to drugs activated in the body.

Clinical Applications of Pharmacokinetic Principles

The different Pharmacokinetic principles, processes and knowledge can be applied for the benefit of all in different manners:

1. To prolong the action of drugs:

    - Via Absorption :

        By prolonging drug absorption from the site of administration, the total action of the drug is enhanced for a long time duration.

        In the Oral drug administration, various dosage forms like spansules, sustained release tablets serve the function. In these preparations, drug particles are coated with different materials which step by step deliver drug particles to the recipient body. At least drug duration of action increases by 4-8 hours.

        In Parenteral drug administration, depot preparations or injections are used s.c. or i.m. (benzathine penicillin, insulin, progestins), biodegradable implants are used.. All these efforts result in elongating drug action from a few days to several months or even years.

Transdermal Drug Delivery patches are also a good method to increase drug duration of action .E.g. GTN

- Via PPB:

By preparing drug analogues which can bind to plasma proteins to a great extent, then these are slowly released and their duration of action is elongated. E.g. Sulfadoxine

- Via metabolism of drugs:

By small changes and efforts like adding ethinyl group to estradiol (ethinyl estradiol), by using drug inducing and inhibiting mechanisms like ritonavir stimulates levels of lopinavir, etc, such adoption of different techniques and changing metabolism to slight extent can make the drug long acting.

- Via Drug Excretion:

By suppressing tubular secretion of drugs with competing substances like probenecid, the duration of action of object drugs like ampicillin, penicillin, etc can be increased.

- Benefits of prolonging drug action duration:
    - Reduces drug administration frequency.

- Better patient compliance (due to less dosing frequency, doses are not missed, always remembered)

- Great fluctuations in plasma drug concentration are not seen, better drug monitoring is achieved

- Drug effects can be prolonged overnight - no sleep disturbances. E.g. Antiasthmatic drugs.

2. Target Drug Delivery devices

These are the novel means to specifically target, localise and deliver the drug for longer duration to the target sites in the body.

- Liposomes -Lecithin is sonicated and made into unilamellar or bilamellar small vesicles (60-80 nM). These are injected I.v. , then taken up by RE cells of the spleen and liver, the drug is released and shows response. E.g. liposomal Amphotericin B finds use in Kala Azar.

- Implants- Implants are coated with drugs and placed in the organ, where they deliver drugs for a long time duration. E.g. Intra Uterine Contraceptive Devices (IUCD) containing Progestins deliver drugs upto 5 years. Stents impregnated with Antithrombotic drugs are used to prevent restenosis and also failure of angioplasty (balloon angioplasty).

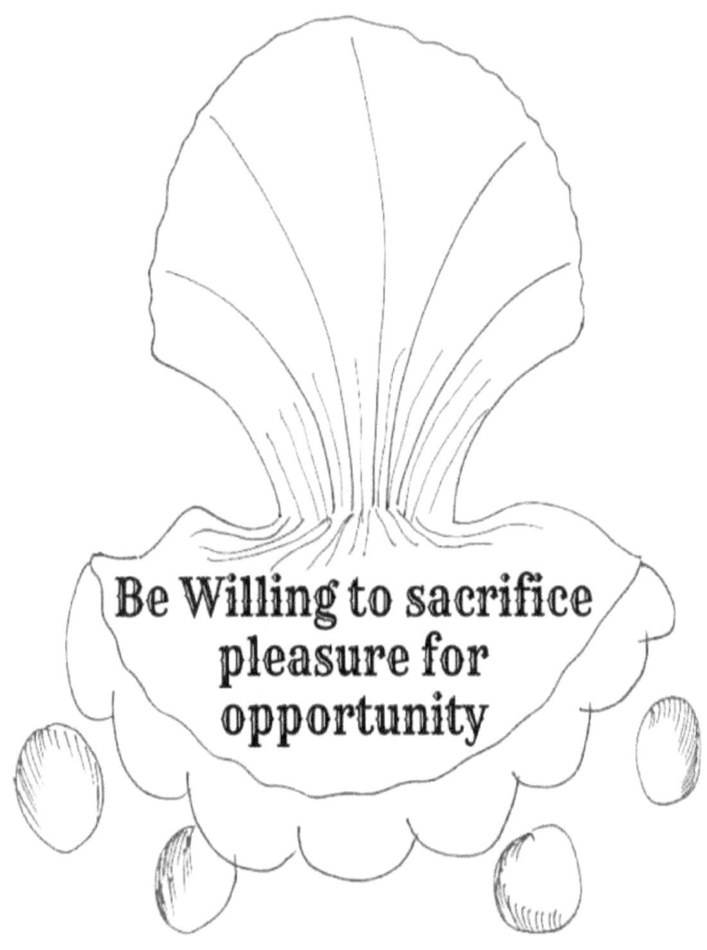
Be Willing to sacrifice
pleasure for
opportunity

Chapter 4

Pharmacodynamics at a Glance-1

KEY FEATURES

- *Introduction to Pharmacodynamics*

- *Drug mechanisms*

- *Receptor Pharmacology*

Definition:

The study of effects of drugs with complete description about drug mechanism, especially details of action-effect and dose-effect relations and alteration of these parameters all-inclusively is termed as Pharmacodynamics.

Drug Action Mechanism:

- Stimulation refers to increased activity of specialised cells (stimulation of heart by adrenaline, stimulation of intestinal smooth muscle by Acetylcholine)

- Depression refers to selective impediment of special cell activity (Acetylcholine depresses heart and Adrenaline depresses intestinal motility)

- Some drug actions are a product of their physical or chemical characteristics.(Antacids neutralise gastric HCl, charcoal adsorbs toxins when activated, Chelating agents like EDTA forms complex with heavy metals)

Drug acts on different large molecular sites (mainly protein in nature):

- Ion channels:

  These are selective protein moieties, composed of ions. Specific signals direct the drugs to bind to ion channels. If binding is direct, they are known as *Ligand gated channels,* sometimes they are *Voltage gated channels,* while if G-Proteins are a medium, they are *G-Protein channels.*

- Enzymes:

  Enzymes act as catalysts and influence different reactions. The effect can be enhanced or depressed by the drugs. This is done by *Enzyme Induction* or *Enzyme Inhibition.* Latter can be Competitive or Non Competitive.

  - Enzyme Induction- An enhancement in activity of enzyme as a result of more synthesis is termed as *Enzyme Induction.* Amongst the different parameters, kM is increased and Vmax decreases. E.g., Failure of Oral contraceptives occurs due to Enzyme induction by Rifampicin administered simultaneously.

- Competitive Enzyme Inhibition- There is structural similarity amongst the drug and enzyme and a competition occurs for binding site, result being no/damaged product. A novel equilibrium is achieved , hence this process is also termed as the *Equilibrium type* of Inhibition. As far as the parameters are concerned, kM increases, Vmax is unchanged.

  If there is *Non Equilibrium* Enzyme Inhibition, then drugs cannot displace the enzyme as the bonds are very strong (covalent bonds) E.g. phenoxybenzamine binds and inhibits alpha adrenergic receptors non selectively and irreversibly. Amongst the parameters, kM is increased and Vmax is reduced.

- Non Competitive Enzyme Inhibition- In this type of Enzyme inhibition, the sites of binding of drug and enzyme are separate, not same. The mechanism is the change in conformation of the enzyme , hence it loses its activity. Amongst the parameters, kM is unchanged, Vmax is reduced. E.g. Inhibitory effect of Cyanide on cytochrome oxidase , inhibitory effect of Sildenafil on Phosphodiesterase-5.

- Membrane transporters:

These serve as carriers of many substances/drugs across the membranes. This movement can be in two directions, firstly along the concentration gradient, secondly, against it. The latter requires energy to occur.

There are three main types of membrane transporters.

- ABC Transporters- They are primary active transporters, transporting the substances mainly out of the cell membrane.. Main substrates for these are lipids, ions, small molecules, sterols, large peptide drugs. If their number increases in states of malignancy, then they critically work to develop multi drug resistance as the therapeutic drugs are pumped out faster than their entry into the cell.

- P-Type ATPases- Theses are in fact the enzyme family which via primary active transport pumps cations out of membranes.E.g. Calcium ATPases, Na-K-ATPases

- Solute Carrier Family (SLC)-This consist of transporters utilising secondary active transport and facilitated diffusion. Their sites are intracellular as well as on cell membranes.E.g. are biogenic amine transporters (SERT, DAT). Therapeutically, inhibitors of SLC transporters are used for many brain and cognitive disorders like depression (SERT Inhibitors), Parkinson's disease (DAT Inhibitors)

- Receptors:

Definition:

Receptors are regulatory macromolecules involved in chemical signalling not only within the cells but also in between the cells. Their site of location may be on the cell membrane surface or inside the cytoplasm. Once activated, regulation of a variety of cellular biochemical processes (enzyme activity, DNA transcription, ion conductance,etc.) occur directly or indirectly. These receptors control the activity of effectors like protein structures, channels, enzymes, transporters, etc.)

Types of Receptors:

Large variety of receptors have been discovered, identified and obtained via Molecular cloning, isolation, etc. Those which bind to the ligand and act via transmitters, signal molecules, hormones, etc are called *Physiological receptors*. E.g. Insulin, adrenergic, histaminergic receptors. On the other hand, *Drug* receptors need no ligands, E.g. Benzodiazepine receptor. *Orphan* receptors are those for which no endogenous ligands are discovered.

On the basis of different criteria, receptors are classified. Traditionally and pharmacologically, the potency of agonists and antagonists forms the basis of classification (alpha and beta receptors). Affinity of binding ligand (serotonin receptors), Distribution in different tissues (beta 1 in heart and beta 2 in lungs), Difference in signalling pathway (GABA-a is ligand gated ion channel while GABA-b is G-Protein receptor) are other basis of receptor classification. Molecular cloning has helped to identify many types and subtypes of receptors.

Function of Receptors:

Receptors serve manifold functions like carrying regulatory signals from one direction to the other of effector cells, signal enhancement and coordination of intracellular and extracellular signals and maintain a healthy state of balance in between various biochemical and physiological functions. With higher degree of adaptation to long and short duration alterations in the environment, receptors assure their consistency and stability and proper functioning.

Receptor Theory:

This was propounded by Clark in 1937, the main idea of which can be stated as, Interaction between Drug and Receptor occurs , there is formation of Drug receptor complex and effect is produced.

$$\mathbf{D+R=DR\text{-----------}E(effect)}$$

- Affinity-Its the binding capability of a drug to the receptor. It is directly proportional to the drug concentration and related number of DR complexes formed.

- Efficacy-After binding, the ability of a drug to produce a response or in other words a functional change in receptor is known as *Efficacy* or *Intrinsic Activity*. It has a numerical value ranging from -1 to +1.

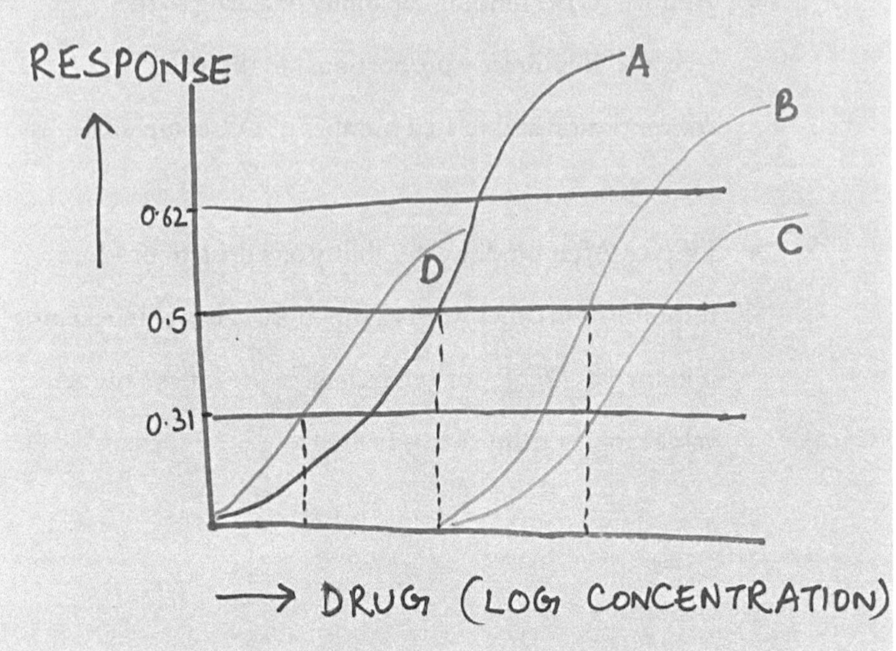

Fig 9. Drug Potency and Drug Efficacy

(Drug B is less potent but equally efficacious as Drug A

Drug C is less potent and less efficacious than Drug A

Drug D is more potent than drugs A,B, and C

but less efficacious than drugs A & B,

And equally efficacious than Drug C)

- Agonists- Substances binding to the receptor and bringing about functional change and response. Hence they possess both Affinity and Efficacy (IA=+1).E.g., morphine, adrenaline, codeine, fentanyl.

- Antagonists-Substances which hinder binding action of an Agonist to the receptor and prevent the functional response from occurring, but totally non functional on their own are called Antagonists. Hence they possess Affinity, but no Intrinsic Activity (IA=0) E.g., Haloperidol, Naltrexone, Phenoxybenzamine.

- Partial Agonist-Substances which on binding to the receptor activate and produce suboptimal action, on the other hand they behave as full antagonists in the presence of full agonist. Hence they have Affinity and submaximal Efficacy (IA between 0 and 1), E.g., Buspirone, buprenorphine, aripiprazole.

- Inverse Agonists-After binding to the receptor, thi substance produces response opposite to that of the Agonist, hence known as Inverse Agonist, it has Affinity, but Efficacy is in negative sign (IA= -1)
  These substances exhibit *Constitutive Activation,* i.e. possess little activity in complete absence of an Agonist(Basal state). E.g., Beta carboline is inverse agonist at Benzodiazepine receptor, nearly all H1 and H2 antihistamines are shown to be inverse agonists.

Dual State Receptor model:

- It is assumed that a receptor exists in two forms or states which can interchange.

  The active form is designated as "Ra" while inactive form is designated as "Ri".

  Generally these are found in balanced state, rather upto slight level, inactive state is dominant. Little or Nil constitutive activation is shown.

- Agonists bind actively to "Ra" form, equilibrium shifts and response is generated.

- Competitive antagonist binds to both forms, no equilibrium shifts and no response is generated.

- Partial agonist generates submaximal response as only little more of it binds to "Ra" than "Ri" , hence little shift of equilibrium occurs.

- Inverse agonists bind actively to "Ri", equilibrium shifts more towards "Ri" and opposite response is generated.

- Constitutive activation is the response generation even when no agonist is present. It is exhibited by adrenergic beta 1, histamine H2, benzodiazepine receptor etc.

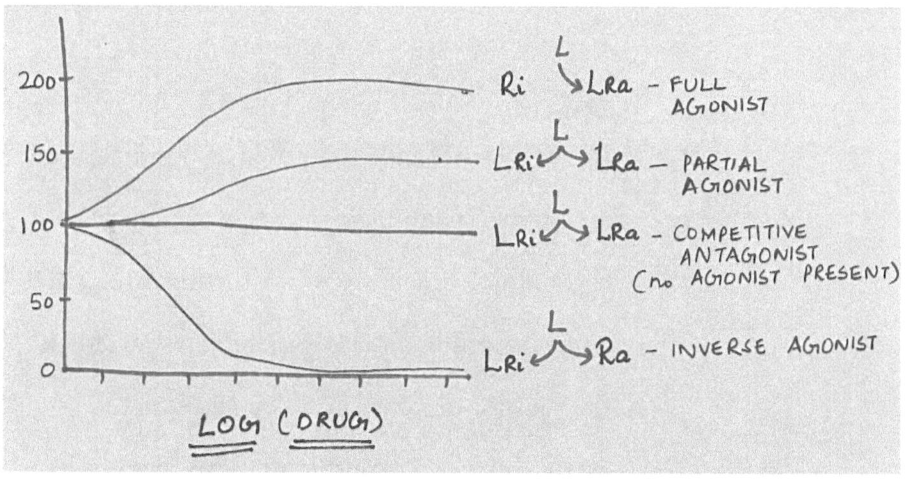

Fig 10. Classification of Ligands on basis of Dual Nature of Receptor (L=Ligand, Ri=Inactive state of Receptor, Ra=Active state of Receptor)

Signalling Transduction Pathways:

Drug action is the result of binding of either Agonist or Antagonist with the receptor which may or may not bring about a conformational change in the receptor . On the other hand, *Drug effect* is the consequence of stepwise drug action that is represented as a final change in biological function.

DRUG ACTION -----LEADS TO --------DRUG EFFECT

- G-Protein coupled receptor:

  Cell membrane receptors and effectors

  (enzymes/transporter) are linked via G-Proteins

★ Structure of G-Protein coupled receptor:

It is a large molecule composed of 7-alpha helical membrane spanning segments of Amino acids , hydrophobic in nature which further extend in 3-3 each extracellular and intracellular loops. In this, the Agonist binding site lies in loops on the extracellular end. Another site at the cytosolic end binds the G-Proteins.

G-Proteins are composed of basic three subunits, alpha, beta, gamma. Their inter-associations decide the state of the receptor. When GDP is bound to alpha subunit, the receptor is in Inactive state. When GDP gets displaced by GTP, alpha subunit carrying GTP dissociates from beta-gamma subunits and the receptor is said to be in Active or state. This may further stimulate or inhibit a response. Alpha subunit contains GTPase activity, this hydrolyses GTP back to GDP in some time. Alpha subunit once detached, binds back to beta-gamma dimer and vicious cycle ensues. A regulating protein, RGS monitors the rate of GTP hydrolysis

Different forms of G-Protein receptors are identified like Gs, Gi, Gq, etc. For G-Protein coupled receptor to operate, there are major three effector pathways:

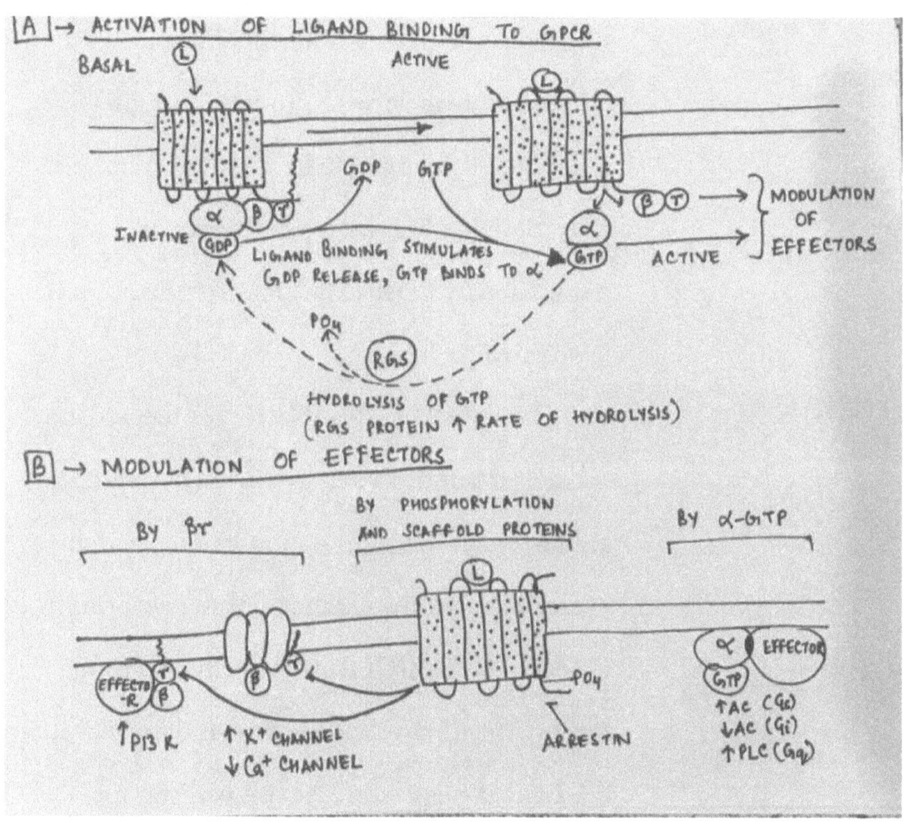

Fig 11. G-Protein Coupled Receptor Activation & Effector pathways

★ Adenylyl cyclase:cAMP Pathway:

Adenylyl cyclase is activated, it enhances storage of cAMP, which is the second messenger. cAMP works mainly through Protein kinase A (PKa). PKa alters the state of different effectors like enzymes, transporters to produce responses like generation of impulse in heart, smooth muscle relaxation, lipolysis etc. cAMP action is terminated by PDEs (Phosphodiesterases) , it is hydrolysed to 5-AMP.

NOTE- cGMP (cyclic GMP) is another second messenger but restricted to few sites like intestine, kidney, etc. It mediates responses like smooth muscle relaxation and salt and water absorption. Guanylyl cyclase (GC) exists in either cytosolic form or membrane bound form and none of these is GPCR. Drugs acting via this pathway are Sodium nitroprusside and Glyceryl trinitrate.

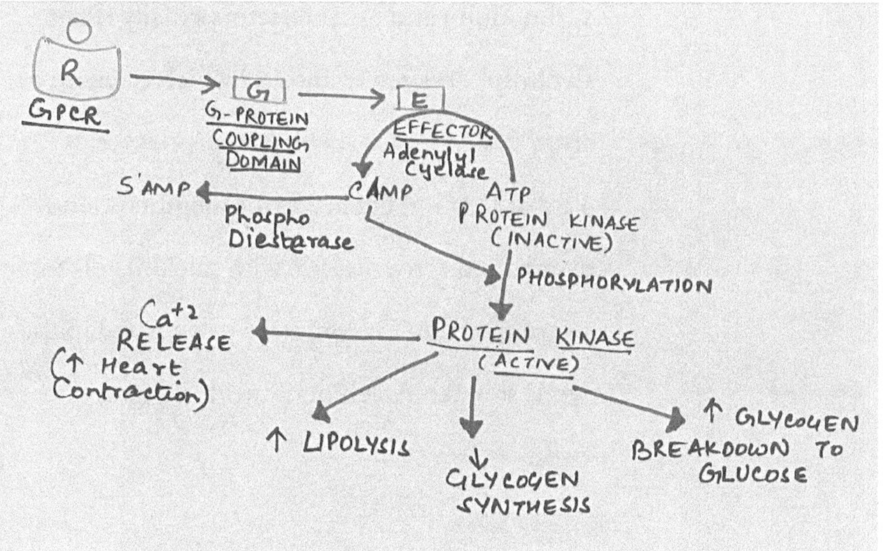

Fig 12. Adenylyl cyclase-cAMP Pathway of GPCR

★ Phospholipase C:IP3 DAG Pathway:

GTP carrying alpha subunit activates

Phospholipase c-beta. (PLcb) which hydrolyses

PhosphatidylInositol 4,5 Bisphosphate (PIP2),

this generates two second messengers namely,

Inositol 1,4,5 trisphosphate (IP3) and

Diacylglycerol (DAG)

Fate of IP3 is- being water soluble, it helps in

release of Calcium in the cytosol through

Endoplasmic reticulum. Calcium is acting as the

third messenger here. It performs its functions via

Calmodulin and other effectors.Finally IP3 is dephosphorylated to Inositol which is reused to form PIP2.

Fate of DAG- it lies inside the membrane and assigns and activates PKc with calcium aid. Some portion of DAG is converted to phospholipids, while some to Arachidonic acid and its action ends.

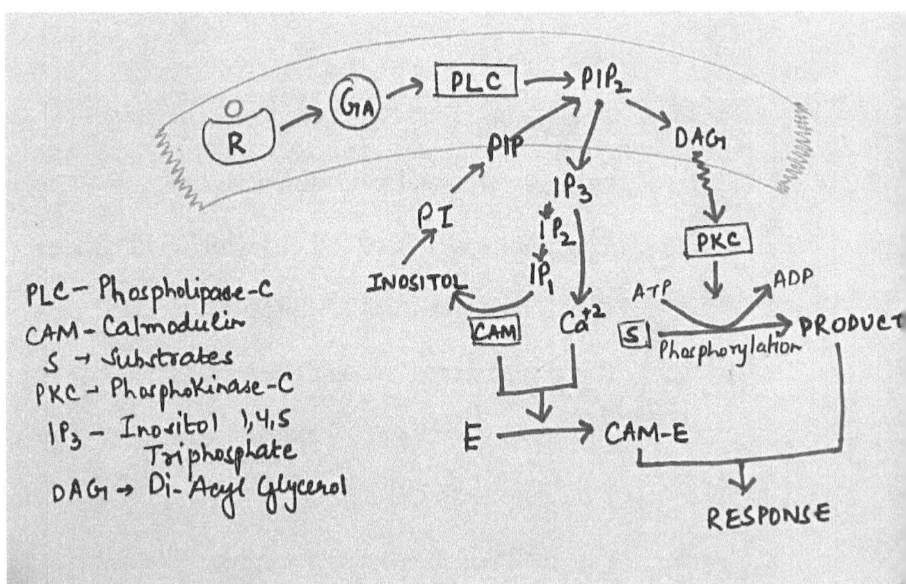

Fig 13. Phospholipase C-IP3-DAG Pathway of GPCR

★ Regulation of Channels:

Different forms of G-Proteins like Gs, Gi, Gq, etc. in activated state can directly affect the Ion channels of Calcium, Potassium. No second messengers are required for response generation. To be specific Gs opens calcium channels in heart and muscles, Gi inhibit calcium channels in and around nerves , while opens potassium channels of heart. Beta-gamma dimer is the operating hero in this story of Ion channel regulation. These may be exhibited as different kinds of responses in the body, inotropy, release of transmitter, relaxation of smooth muscles.

- Enzyme linked Tyrosine kinase receptors:
Structurally, there is a large ligand binding end linked to intracellular subunits which possess enzyme activity (Protein kinase or Guanylyl cyclase). Linking is via transmembrane helical peptide bonds. In most of the cases, Protein kinase moiety is *Receptor Tyrosine kinases*

(RTKs) E.g. Insulin, various growth factors, Anticancer drugs, etc.

As far as mechanism is concerned, In unbound form, the receptor is inactive, Once the hormone binds, two receptors unite to form a dimer. This leads to conformational change which further appreciates autophosphorylation of tyrosine residues, one over the other. Dimerization also affects receptor internalization, lysosomal degradation and down regulation. Finally affinity for protein substrates carrying SH2 domains is increased, they are phosphorylated, released in a cascade form finally generating responses like cell growth and differentiation. IP3 and DAG are too generated which affect the responses.

Generally responses via these receptors occur within a few minutes to a few hours.

NOTE- If there is Guanylyl cyclase substituting Protein Kinase, cGMP is generated as a second messenger which further leads to response cascade. E.g. ANP (Atrial natriuretic peptide)

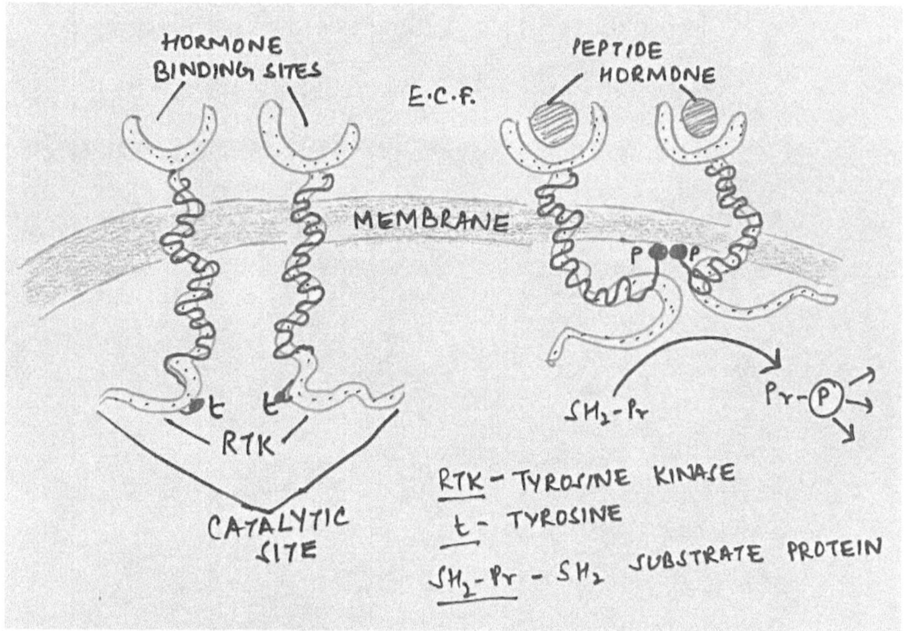

Fig 14. Tyrosine kinase enzyme linked receptor functioning

- JAK-STAT binding Transmembrane Receptors:
  Drug induces formation of receptor dimers, changes in conformation, increased affinity for a different type of cytosolic protein kinase namely JAK (Janus Kinase), this type of receptor lacks intrinsic catalytic activity. After being bound, JAK is activated, it phosphorylates the receptor residues. These tyrosine residues catch hold of STAT (Signal Transducer and Activation of transcription), a free protein entity, whis is too phosphorylated.

Phosphorylated STAT dimerizes in pairs and regulates gene transcription in the nucleus and response is generated. E.g. Prolactin, growth hormone, cytokines, etc.

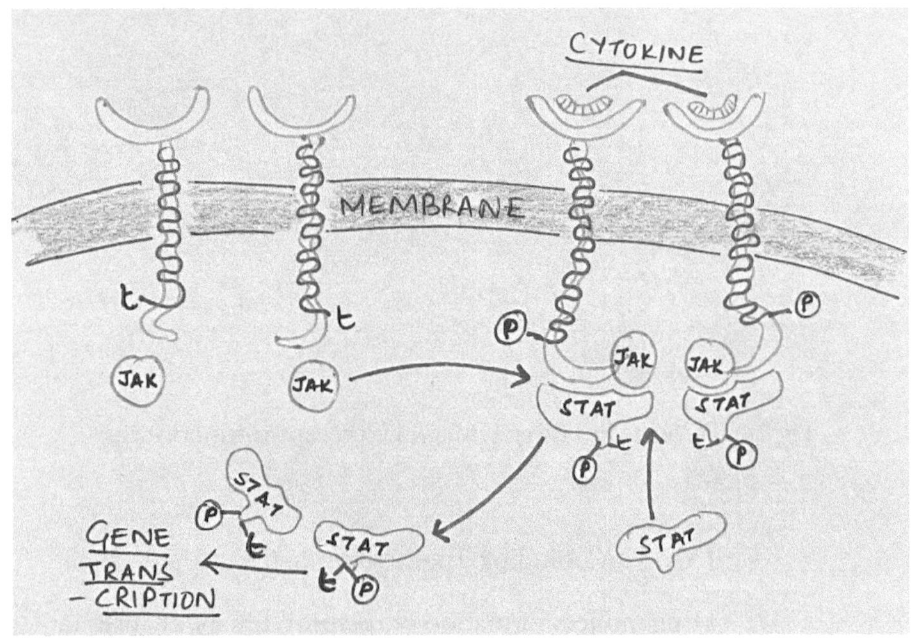

Fig 15. Transmembrane JAK-STAT Binding receptor functioning

- Nuclear receptors:

  These receptors are present inside the cell , either in cytoplasm or in the nucleus. Lipid soluble drugs enter the cell and bind to these receptors. In normal state, the receptor stays bound to HSP-90 protein, which is released on binding of drug (hormone) to the receptor. Now dimerization of the receptor occurs and the DNA binding segment is folded into active form. The dimer binds other co-activators/co-repressors inside the nucleus which highly affects the function of genes. This whole complex binds to its respective hormone response element (specific DNA Sequence) and accordingly either stimulates or depresses to step up or step down specific mRNA synthesis. Further specific proteins are synthesised to affect target cells or activity. E.g. Steroidal hormones, vit D, vit A, etc. This type of response effectuation vi aNuclear receptors is very slow in time duration, and takes a few hours to accomplish the desired results. Proteins have slow turnover, the effect prolongs even after hormone is excreted.

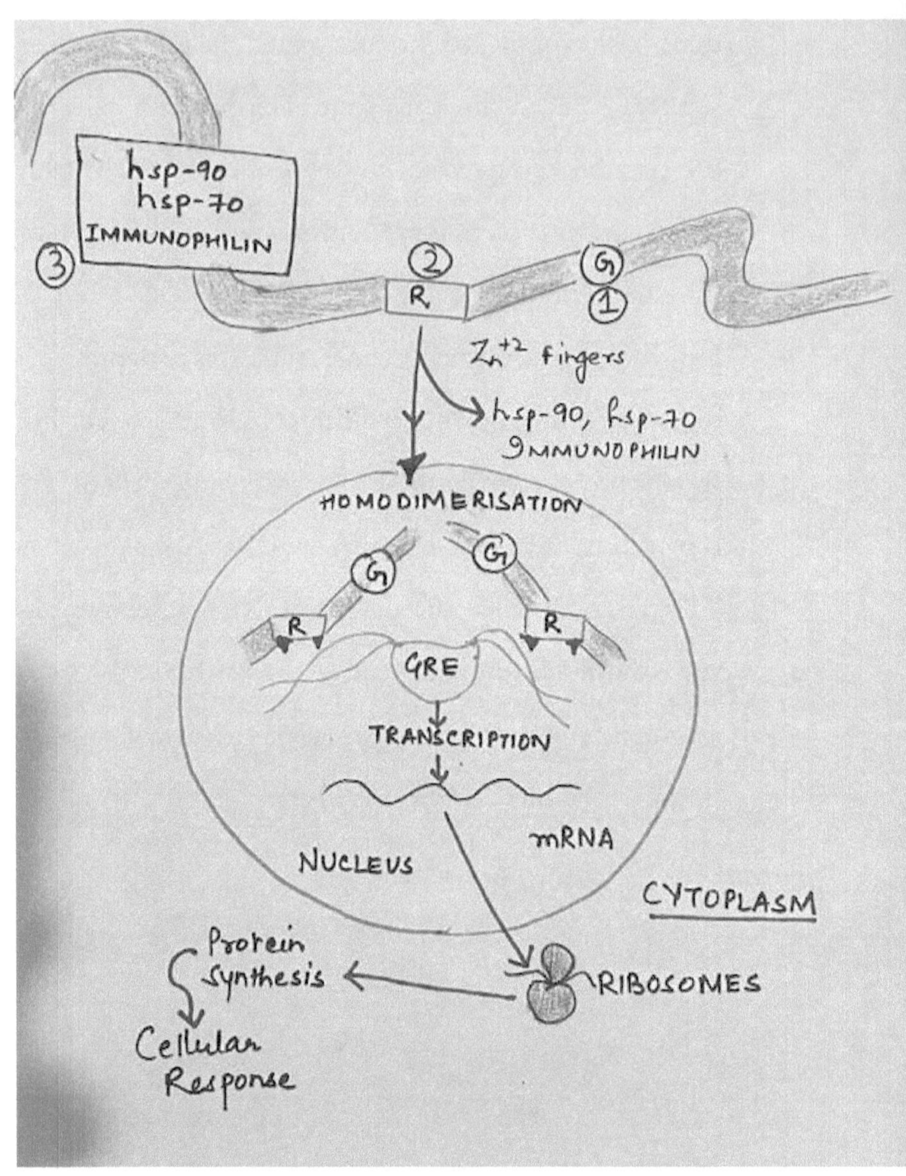

Fig 16. Intracellular (intranuclear) receptor operating mechanism (Glucocorticoid receptor example through which gene transcription and further protein synthesis occurs)

Receptor Regulation:

Efficacy and receptor concentration are a function of the activity of the body and various pathophysiological mechanisms undergoing. All this decides the level of sensitivity and also supersensitivity of receptors (Occurring due to agonist deprivation of receptors for long periods). E.g. in case of sudden withdrawal of drug like clonidine, there occurs receptor unmasking or proliferation or best known as *"Up Regulation"* which enhances response magnitude manifold.

On the contrary, if there is regular and continuous stimulation of receptors via Agonists, there arises a state of refractoriness or desensitisation , resulting in decreased response magnitude. E.g. Continuous administration of levodopa in parkinsonism, gradually declines response efficacy.

"Down regulation" refers to decreased magnitude of receptors either due to decreased production or increased destruction. It takes a lot of time to turn to normal , around weeks to months. E.g. Some tyrosine kinases exhibit such a response.

Another way to classify desensitisation is either Heterologous (Exposure to one agonist decreases response to all agonists via various receptors producing similar effect) or Homologous

(Exposure to one agonist decreases response to all agonists of same receptors) . GPCRs are apt examples for both types.

Spare Receptors:

Generally complete drug response is observed even when less than 100% of receptors are occupied. The rest of the unoccupied receptors serve simply as reserve and are known as "Spare receptors". Spare Receptors are the receptors that exist in excess of those required to produce a full effect. E.g Blocking of Acetylcholine with a toxin shows effect only when 50% of receptors are bound to toxin, 1% of LH receptor binding to Leydig cells shows great level of steroidogenesis.

These can be experimentally exposed with Irreversible Antagonists and further by showing that maximal response can be generated with high agonist concentrations. E.g. Insulin receptors (about 90% act as spare receptors)

Receptor related diseases and Non Receptor Mechanisms:

Receptor related diseases are Myasthenia Gravis (antibodies develop against cholinergic nicotinic receptors at motor end plate), Insulin resistant diabetes, testicular feminisation (due to androgen receptor insensitivity), etc.

Apart from acting on receptors, drug may exhibit responses via:

- Chemical actions- Neutralisation reactions (antacids, anticoagulants ike heparin), Chelation (chelating agents like EDTA, Dimercaprol, Penicillamine, deferoxamine trap Pb, As, Fe, Cu, Hg), Ion Exchangers like cholestyramine (anion exchange resins) exchanges Cl ions from bile salts and help lower down cholesterol.

- Physical Action- Astringents (they precipitate and denature mucosal proteins like tannic acid), Demulcents (Coat the inflamed surface and provide soothing effect like pectin, menthol), Protectives (dusting powders), Adsorbents (Kaolin, Simethicone), Osmosis (Magnesium sulphate as purgative) and Saturation in biophase (GAs saturate cell biophase of CNS and disrupt the function)

- Through Antibody formation or Placebo action- Vaccines (cholera, smallpox) induce antibody formation while starch or lactose act as placebo (Pharmacologically inert compound which brings about relief in subjective symptoms due to psychological problems of anxiety, stress, etc. in a placebo rector, the patient is termed as *Placebo*)

- By false incorporation method- In sulfa drugs, methotrexate, such a process is seen, these drugs falsely enter the synthetic process in place of PABA and makes the resultant compound non functional . This is a bacteriostatic action, while in case of methotrexate, it is a cytotoxic action by hindering DNA production.

- Protoplasmic poisons and Gene function alteration- Some germicides, antiseptics (phenol) serve as protoplasmic poisons to kill bacteria. Anticancer drugs are a product of gene function alteration like Farnesyl transferase (inhibits ras-modifying enzyme) reverses cancerous effects of ras-oncogene and Tyrosine kinase Inhibitors block oncogenic kinases.

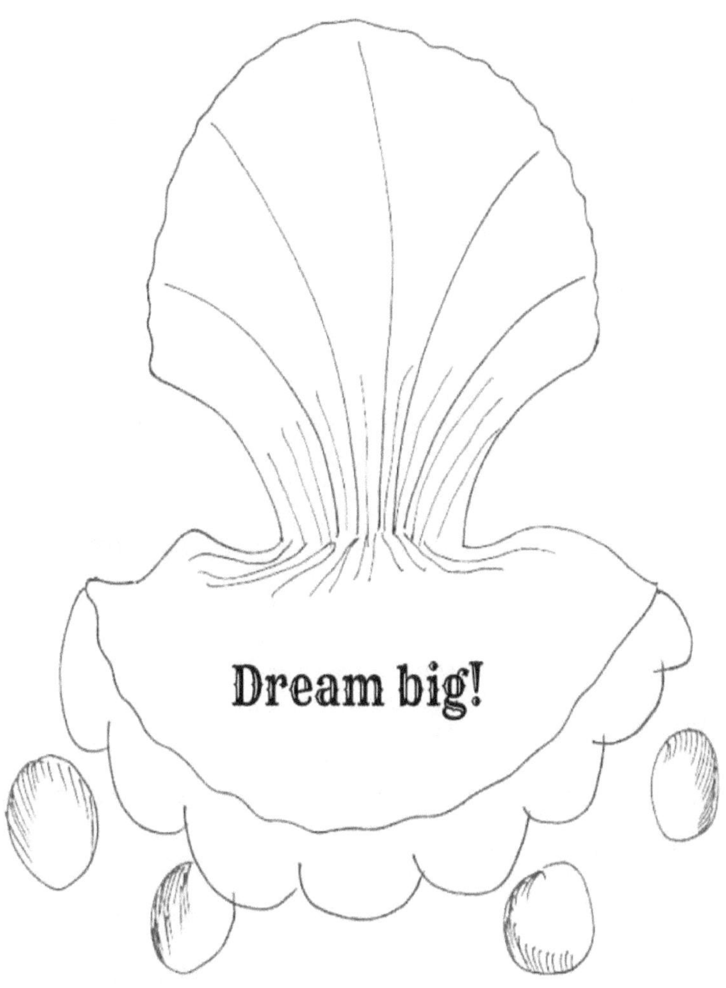

Dream big!

Chapter 5

Pharmacodynamics at a Glance-2

KEY FEATURES

- *Dose Response Relationship*
- *Definitions*
- *Drug Synergism*
- *Drug Antagonism*

Once a drug is administered via a systemic route, we obtain some important relations via graphs.

Dose response curve is a graphical relation of drug dose given (X-axis) and drug effect (Y-axis). It has two main components:

1. Dose- plasma concentration relation
2. Plasma concentration response relation

The concentration response relation for drugs may turn out to be Graded or Quantal in nature.

- Quantal DRC-

    It can give an idea of changing response patterns as the drug dose increases in different individuals. Quantal concentration-effect curve is drawn for drugs exhibiting "All or None response", (antiemetic stops vomiting or not). Its used to determine ED50 and LD50 values

- Graded DRC-

    A graded concentration-effect curve is achieved when effects are determined on a continuous scale (reduction in blood pressure) ; they effectively define the relation between extent of response and dose value , effectively signifying Drug Action.

Normally, with increase in drug dose the response also increases upto certain level, then it starts fading and the Graph we get is "Rectangular Hyperbola".

If the same response is plotted on log scale , the graph obtained is "Sigmoid" in shape and also a linear relation amongst log value of dose and value of response is observed significantly in the mid 1/3rd zone. To summarise, response increases exponentially with log dose value. The log dose response curve (DRC) enables us to display a large range of doses of drugs and it becomes very easy to study and mark comparisons amongst agonists and antagonists.

We can identify few important parameters:

1. Drug Potency:

    The drug amount required to produce a response is the measure of drug potency. In the DRC (graded dose response curve), it matches to the point on the dose axis. It governs the choice of drug dose. On DRC, it can be identified easily, leftward shifting signifies high potency while rightward shifting signifies less potency.

2. Drug Efficacy:

The maximum response that can be obtained by a drug is the measure of its efficacy. In the DRC, it coincides with the maximal height obtained on the graph. Overall it governs the choice of drug as a whole. (more powerful tool than drug potency).

3. DRC Slope:

It is also a beneficial parameter, if it goes steep, it explains that a little increase in drug dose will actually make a great difference in drug response, hence drug dose varies from person to person. While that is true opposite for flat dose where standardisation of drug dose can be done over a group or population of masses.(Drugs with steep DRC are CNS depressants while Antihypertensives like hydrochlorothiazide have flat DRC)

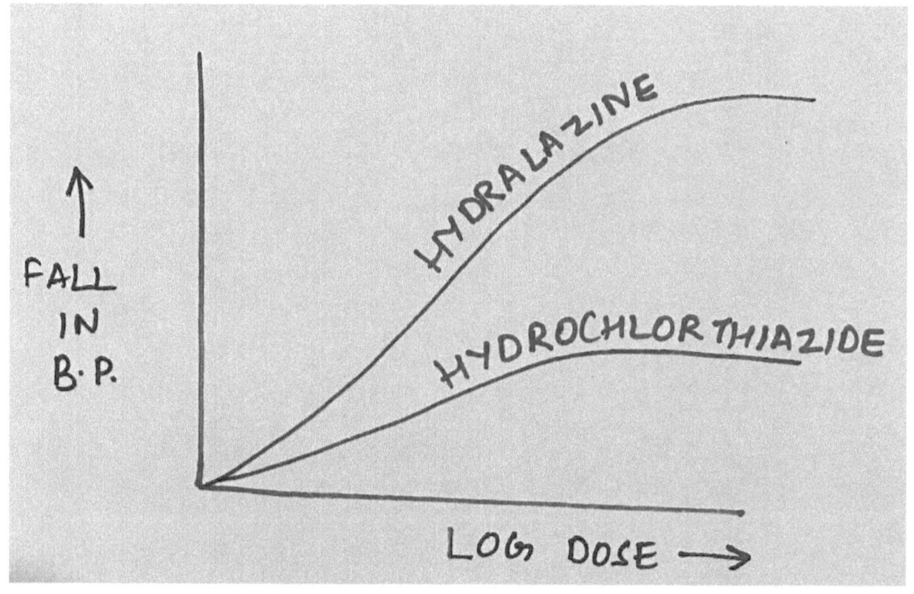

Fig 17. Flattening of Dose Response Curve (DRC)

(Example of two drugs for blood pressure is shown and efficacy compared)

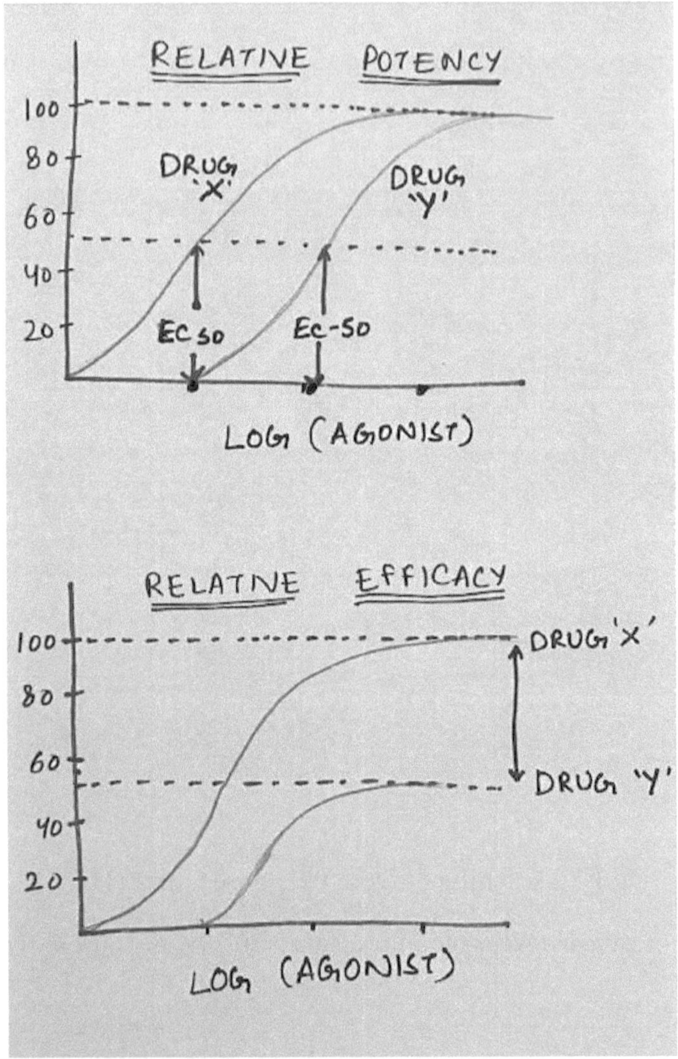

Fig 18. In graph-1, comparative potency of two drugs X & Y is compared,

The rightward shift shows decreased potency.

In graph-2, comparative efficacy of two drugs is shown,

flattening of DRC shows decreased efficacy

4. Drug Selectivity:

Drug Selectivity is measured by the extent of distance between different DRCs (for different responses) of drug, it clearly shows drug selectivity, more the distance more the selectivity of action.

5. Therapeutic Index:

Therapeutic index is defined as the ratio of LD50 to ED50.

Therapeutic Index or Drug Safety margin is obtained by measure of distance amongst the DRCs of therapeutic response and Side effects of drug.

Formula to calculate Therapeutic Index is :

Therapeutic Index (TI)= Median Lethal dose (LD50)/ Median Effective Dose (ED50)

- Median Effective dose (ED50) :

  It is the dose which shows the response in half (50%) of the participants.

- Median Lethal Dose (LD50):

  It is the dose which is lethal to half (50%) of the participants.

6. Therapeutic Window:

It is a "*Therapeutic range*" of doses determined or lying in between least value of possible therapeutic responses at one end and highest value of adverse response tolerated on the other end. This varies from person to person.

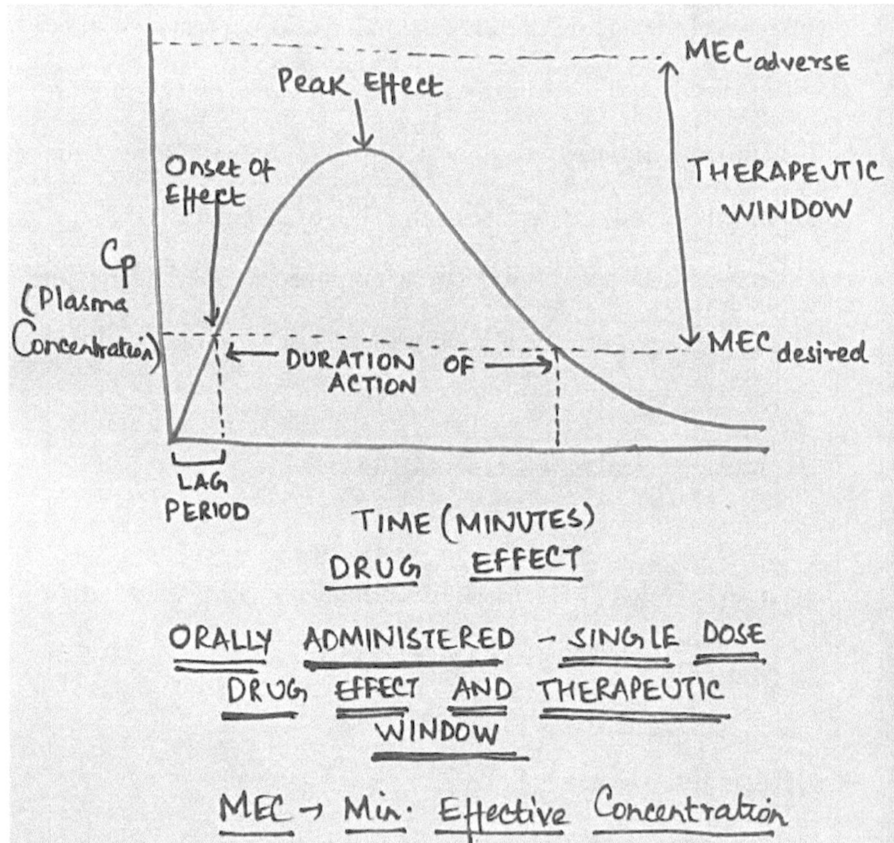

Fig 19. Therapeutic Window illustration
(MEC=Minimum Effective Concentration)

7. Drug Specificity:

It is defined by a variety of possible effects shown by the drug. A drug can produce a single effect or many different kinds of responses depending upon the number of receptors it acts upon and also on the extent of distribution of the receptors in the body. Some specific drugs are Atropine (muscarinic receptor antagonist), Cimetidine (H2 receptor antagonist) and non specific drug examples include Phenothiazine (it blocks D2 dopamine, alpha-adrenergic and muscarinic receptors)

Synergism and Antagonism of Drugs

Administration of more than one drug simultaneously may exhibit no effect or may exhibit their interaction with each other in mainly two forms:

1. Synergism:

It refers to escalation of response of one drug with the help of another drug when given simultaneously. It may further be classified as:

a) Additive:

Both the drugs act in the same uniform direction and their net response is summation of individual drug responses.(Aspirin and acetaminophen show analgesia and blood thinning, Glibenclamide and metformin show added hypoglycemic effect)

A+B=Response of A+Response of B

b) Potentiation (Supra Additive):

Both the drugs act in the same uniform direction and their net response is more than simple summation of individual drug responses.(NSAIDs and opioids show improved analgesia in postoperative period,Aspirin and Clopidogrel show much more blood thinning together, Sulfamethoxazole and Trimethoprim show potentiated antimicrobial effect)

A+B>Response of A+Response of B

2. Antagonism:

It refers to decrease or nullification of response of one drug due to another drug.

A+B<Response of A+Response of B

It may be further classified as :

(a) PHYSICAL ANTAGONISM:

It is explained by physical properties of drugs antagonising each other's effects. Charcoal adsorbs alkaloids in case of poisoning.

(b) PHYSIOLOGICAL ANTAGONISM:

Drugs antagonise the same physiological function by acting on different sites or receptors or through different mechanisms. Glucagon and Insulin act opposite to each other in concern of blood sugar level. Action of Histamine and Adrenaline is opposite to each other in concern of Blood pressure.

(c) CHEMICAL ANTAGONISM:

In this , chemical interaction of drugs occurs and the final response is decreased or nullified. Chelating agents (BAL) chemically react with heavy metals like As, Pb, etc. Penicillin G and succinyl chloride antagonise each other chemically when mixed together in an injection.

(d) RECEPTOR ANTAGONISM:

In this, one drug is Agonist and the other is Antagonist and the interaction is quite selective. Receptor antagonism can be of two types:

(a) Competitive antagonism:

In the Equilibrium variety, the chemical structure of both agonist and antagonist is similar, and they compete with each other for the same binding site of the receptor. When Antagonist binds to the receptor, no response is elucidated, the Drc shifts to the right side showing low potency. This interaction is reversible in nature, if a large dose of agonist is administered it will surmount the action of Antagonist.

If a partial agonist is administered, it will show competition and may antagonise the complete Agonist , and along with this, it may exhibit some of its own submaximal response.

(b) Non competitive antagonism:

There is no chemical structural similarity in between Agonist and Antagonist, the latter binds to a site different from that of Agonist, which is known as *"Allosteric site"* , this changes the conformation of Receptor in such a way that it becomes incapable of binding to the Agonist and hence no desired response is produced. As the binding sites differ, surmounting this effect is impossible on increasing the amount of Agonist. There is no direct competition.This type of Antagonism is also called *"Allosteric antagonism"*. DRC of Agonist is flattened showing decreased efficacy as the concentration of Antagonist is increased.

In case of Non equilibrium antagonism, the binding of antagonist and receptor is very strong, most of the times via covalent bonds, then Agonist administration cannot reverse this effect and the DRC curve of agonist shifts to the right side and flattening of DRC also occurs. Hence it is also a type of Non competitive Antagonism. E.g. Phenoxybenzamine acting on alpha receptors and antagonising Adrenaline is a good example of this type of Antagnism.

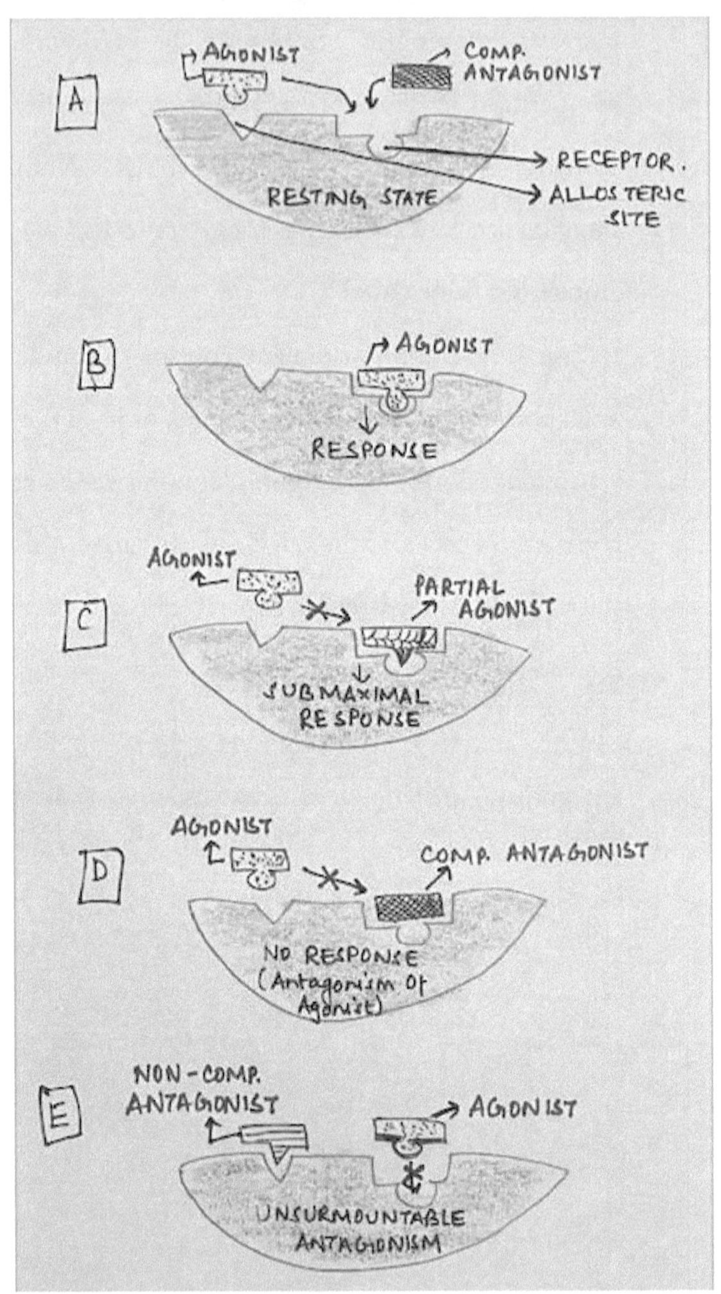

Fig 20. Binding sites of Agonist and Antagonists and Different responses in Different situations

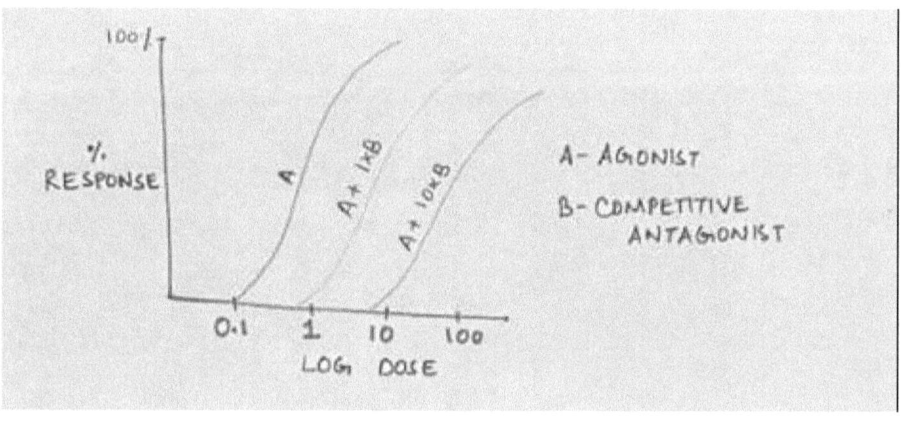

Fig 21. Competitive Antagonism illustration

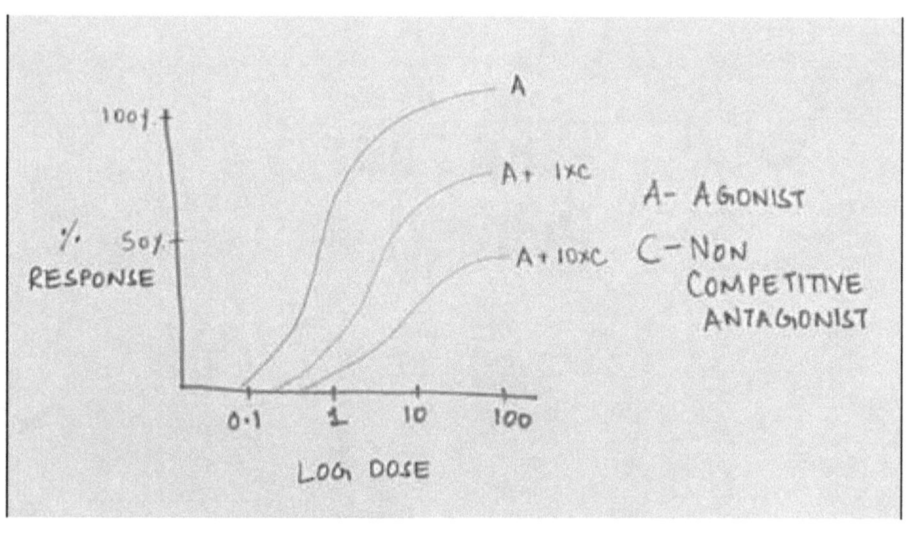

Fig 22 Non Competitive Antagonism illustration.

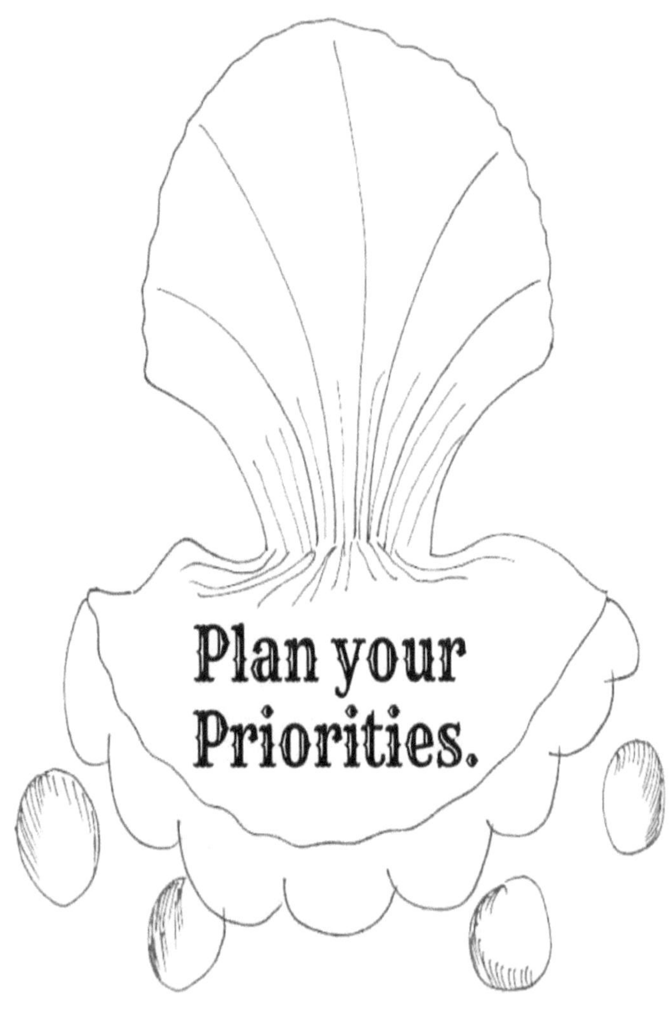

Plan your
Priorities.

Chapter 6

Pharmacogenetics And Pharmacogenomics

KEY FEATURES

- *Definitions*
- *Pharmacogenetic factors*
- *Categories of genetic variations*
- *Identification of new drug pathways*

Definition-

- The study of genetic basis and high degree of responses owing to slight DNA variations for the differences in drug response in different individuals is known as **Pharmacogenetics.**

- Study of many variants in a specific person or larger population group in order to know the influences of genetics over the drug responses is known as **Pharmacogenomics**

The basic goal of both Pharmacogenetics and Pharmacogenomics is to find out apt drugs based on drug effects, then these responses are experimentally checked upon and ensured on the criteria of safety and efficacy and finally these are clinically utilised.

PHARMACOGENETICS

Various factors combinedly work and interact together to finally mould the individual response to a drug. These factors are-

- ☐ Drug factors like dose, route of administration, etc,
- ☐ Environmental factors like diet, toxins, disease, other drugs, etc
- ☐ Clinical factors like indication, organ role, etc
- ☐ Genetic factors

Genes which are involved in the drug effect variability are known as Pharmacogenes and both Pharmacokinetics or Pharmacodynamics can be affected. Mainly pharmacogenes encode drug metabolising enzymes. This drug metabolism can easily be heritable in nature.

As far as origin of Pharmacogenetics is concerned, the description is obtained from times rewind when sir Edward Garrod worked and showed his keen interest in fields of heredity, disease and metabolism. He studied the "Inheritance in Alkaptonuria" and developed the concept of "Inborn errors in metabolism". These inborn errors of metabolism were held responsible for variations in chemical behaviour and also "Chemical Individuality". This became the key foundation stone in the development of "Pharmacogenetics" and "Precision Medicine".

Later, Werner Kalow studied the metabolism of "Succinylcholine" and genetically inherited differences in "Serum Cholinesterase" activity.

CATEGORIES OF GENETIC VARIATIONS

- Population frequency- its larger number decreases the selection pressure
- Base pairs numbers- Single base pairs can be mutated by insertions, deletions, inversions, etc. On the basis of the number of base pairs, there can be - Single nucleotide variants (SNVs) and Copy number Variants (CNVs), the latter being large deletions/duplications.
- Locus in encoded gene
- Effect on protein encoded

Association studies i.e. Genome Wide association studies (GWAS) help to identify many pharmacogenetic variants in "Linkage Disequilibrium" along with functional variants (causal relationship). This pattern is population specific.

"Star Allele" nomenclature of pharmacogenes is quite significant for many Haplotypes. It includes quite a lot of info about several variants across an allele. Standard nomenclature is adopted for drug metabolising enzymes e.g. Poor and Ultrarapid metabolizers.

"Pharmacokinetic alterations" are exhibited when metabolism of drugs is dependent on enzymes or transporters susceptible to functional variability. E.g. drugs metabolised by CYP2D6 like codeine, sparteine, etc. "Pharmacodynamic alterations" can be of two types-

A) Of the Receptor/Target- receptor protein is susceptible to functional variability. E.g. Beta blockers, Aminoglycosides

B) Beyond the Receptor/Target- Wider Biological factors affect drug effects. E.g. G6PD deficiency affecting antimalarial drug response.

"Multigenic Pharmacogenomic traits" are seen when both Pharmacodynamics and Pharmacokinetics phenomenon interplay occurs. One such example is of Warfarin. CYP2C9 enzyme metabolises its active enantiomer. Its effect on the target molecule is encoded by VKORC1 enzyme. Variations in VKORC1 may increase or decrease warfarin resistance. Such variations are common in certain populations which serve as carriers.

Variations in genetics also affect response of Anticancer drugs. HLA alleles are found to be associated with many drug toxicity cases. With their aid, the immune system can markedly recognise foreign and self proteins. Modifications and absence of normal genes can pose risk of many ADRs.

Variety of methods are being adopted to powerfully associate genetic variations and variable responses of drugs. Some examples are are In Silico methods, Single and Multiple experimental approaches, in vitro methods, administration of drugs to genotyped humans and even in mice or similar animal models, generation of Induced pluripotent stem cells (iPSCs) from humans with specific interests and large DNA Biobanks.

GWAS can be used to analyse "Polygenic" drug responses.

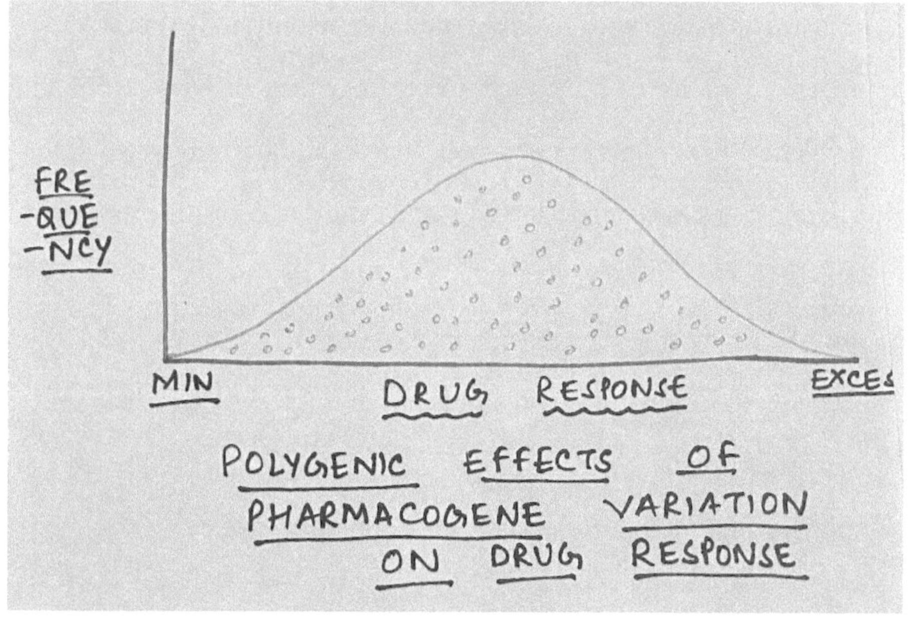

IDENTIFICATION OF NEW DRUG PATHWAYS

Whether in normal physiological states or in pathological states, genetic pathways always hint about new drug receptors or targets. Marketing equally resonates with the genetic support of the drug.

Good examples are of "Alirocumab" and "Evolocumab" targeting PCSK9 - were discovered recently for treatment of lipid disorders.

"Loss-of-function" variants also help by reducing risk for common diseases.

In cystic fibrosis, Ivacaftor and Lumicaftor combination helps be\y improving symptoms.

DNA Biobanks can be applied in a novel manner- Phenome (phenotype of human association with genome) wide Association study (PheWAS) approach can replicate GWAS or discover altogether a new association. This will help to administer novel treatment techniques in targeted populations e.g. Dalcetrapib drug. Targeted anticancer treatments are also benefited.

"Point-of-care" testing allows genotype to be ordered at the time of prescribing, though there are pros and cons of this technique which need to be worked upon.

Employing Pharmacogenetics clinically is still under debate!

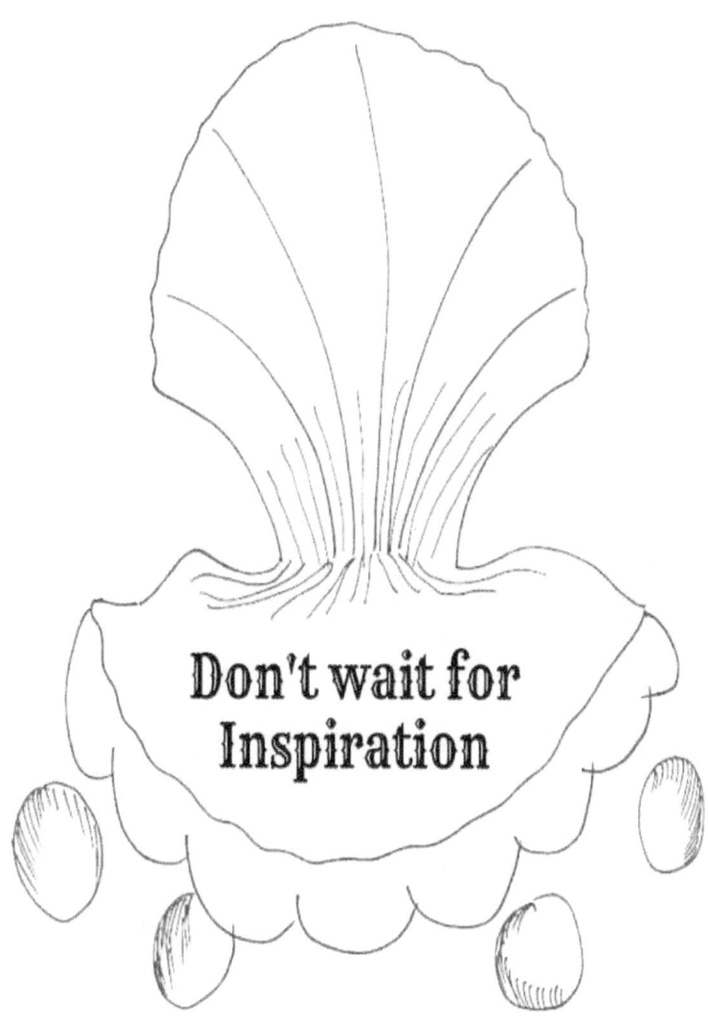

Don't wait for
Inspiration

Chapter 7
Drug Safety and Toxicology

KEY FEATURES

- *Need of Post Marketing Drug Safety*

- *Methods and Actions of Post Marketing Survey*

- *Current challenges and Future prospects of Post marketing drug safety*

- *Drug Toxicity- Introduction and Types*

- *Poisoning- About and Management*

- *Antidotes*

INTRODUCTION

Once the drug is marketed and clinically and therapeutically in use, it has a great potential to exhibit a lot of side effects. Post marketing surveillance helps to learn about the extent and impact of the drug in this direction. This is an effort to improve drug safety.

What is the need of Post Marketing Drug Safety?
The biggest drawback or limitation of Pre Marketing Drug Trials is the satisfactory determination of safety of a drug.

- Number of individuals involved are small, hence rare adverse effects are almost ignored totally. Genetic basis of these ADRs also go unknown

- Time duration of premarketing trials is very short. Hence, long term or chronic side effects go unknown

- A homogenous population is selected for premarketing trials, hence all the detailed, widespread and novel information

- Surrogate endpoints are used often in Premarketing trials which mediate or predict the final clinical endpoints. Some prove excellent, many are misleading also. They are good guides for drug approval.

- Active comparators are not a prominent feature of pre marketing trials. Placebo-controlled studies are permitted and there is great limitation of small sample size. It is very difficult to know well the efficacy and safety of new drugs in comparison to drugs already in vogue in the market.

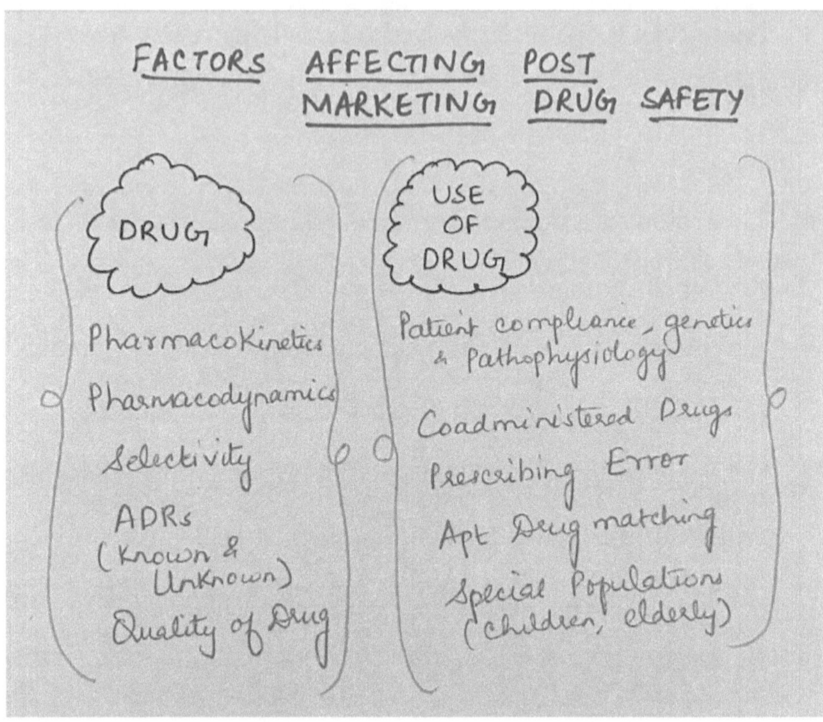

POST MARKETING SURVEILLANCE METHODS AND ACTIONS

- **Case Reports and Spontaneous Adverse Event Reporting Systems-**

  Serious and Important drug safety problems can be recognised and managed especially when drugs are administered in large numbers of people. E.g. Thalidomide tragedy identification and management. The FDA Adverse Event Reporting System (FAERS) in US is very popular and significant.

  Limitation of these tools is the inability to calculate the frequency occurrence of an adverse reaction. Underreporting and heterogeneous pattern of reporting also adversely affects the results. Total number of patients receiving the drug is unknown and Individual case Safety reports are also incomplete. All in all-spontaneous reporting systems cannot identify true events and consequently future evaluation in the form of signalling also Suffers. Good Quality case reports are very important to determine causal relationship between the drug administered and the adverse event.

- **Controlled studies-**

    They have the ability to detect signals arising from case reports and also identify the future drug safety aspects. The "Observational Pharmacoepidemiological studies" collect clinical or insurance data, they are arduous, expensive and quite lengthy in time duration. The drawbacks are made good with "Sentinal system" adopted by FDA in collaboration with many organisations and easy access to electronic data of millions of people. It gives important information about "Drug Utilisation", Signal detection, Signal evaluation, AI use and use of "Real world Data", which has its own pros and cons.

- **Post Marketing Clinical Trials** can effectively evaluate drug safety information and unpredictable side effects. They can be employed to accept/refute a drug safety signal and evaluate its ethical implications.

- The need is not only to gather information but to educate and change the behaviour of the patients and the prescribers.

- **Communication** is an effective tool which is the primary consequence of the reviews of adverse event reports. The posts are regularly updated on the websites to inform everyone regarding safety issues. Adding a "Boxed warning" (black box warning) is an effective and common measure used. Drug Safety Communications (DSCs) are regularly posted on FDA websites. It highly influences the patient and prescriber style and behaviour. Literature review also has manifold effects.

- **Risk Evaluation & Mitigation Strategies (REMS)**. For a particular drug, REMS include medication guides, package inserts, patient register maintenance, regular patient monitoring and follow up, diagnosis, communication and education.

- **Drug withdrawal** from the market, a very drastic and difficult decision - becomes essential when drug risk is too high. E.g.- withdrawal of terfenadine, grepafloxacin, cisapride, etc.

CURRENT AND FUTURE PROSPECTS

- Easy and quick data access is a big challenge in present times. Expensive and difficult access to Medicare data is somewhat relieved by FDA's Sentinal system.

- Great number of Adverse event reports annually equally harbinger challenges and opportunities. Electronic data and AI tools though advanced, have their limitations.

- Inclusion of Pharmacogenetics in Risk Identification and Evaluation is a big challenge but a noteworthy step E.g. in boxed warnings. This approach can aid in determining efficacy and adverse effects of a drug E.g. Mendelian randomisation analysis.

Drug Toxicity: Introduction and Types

KEY FEATURES

- *Definitions*
- *Dose Response Relationships*
- *Effect of Toxicology on Pharmacokinetics- Toxicokinetics*
- *Poisoning- Prevention and Management*
- *Antidotes*

Toxicology- is the study of adverse effects of a variety of chemicals and substances on the living biological system.

Poison- is a substance which causes harmful and deranging effect on the normal physiological system

Clinical Toxicology- the science dealing with undesired effects of pharmaceutical compounds and treatment methods in humans and also with effects and management of poisoning

Generally, toxicology studies are a part and parcel of preclinical animal models testing studies and also in vitro models. Studies related to carcinogens, fertility agents and teratogens are a part of first stage of clinical trials while many and most of the ADRs are discovered in post marketing surveillance.

Dose Response Relationships

In normal measures, DRC are "Graded" in individuals and "Quantal" in a population. In the Graded DRC, response increases with dose increase while in Quantal DRC, population % responding to the drug increases with the dose increase. The latter helps t o determine "Median lethal dose, LD50.

When we have important values and determinants like

ED50 (Median effective dose)- the concentration of a drug at which 50% of population will have desired effect of the drug

and

LD50 (Median lethal dose)- the concentration of the drug at which 50% of population is dead

Then we get

TD50 (Median Toxic dose)- the concentration of drug at which 50% of population will have toxic effect

Accordingly we can evaluate TI (Therapeutic index) in humans and animals as:

In humans- *TI=TD50/ED50*

In animals- *TI= LD50/ED50*

Drugs with low TI have a narrow margin of safety (Digoxin,Warfarin) are to be used with great precaution while drugs with high TI (Penicillin, Ramifentanil) are safe to use.

Median dose, not always effective to evaluate Margin of safety can be alternatively replaced with ED99 for therapeutic effect to be compared to LD1 (animals) or TD1 (humans).

__Margin of Safety= LD1/ED99__

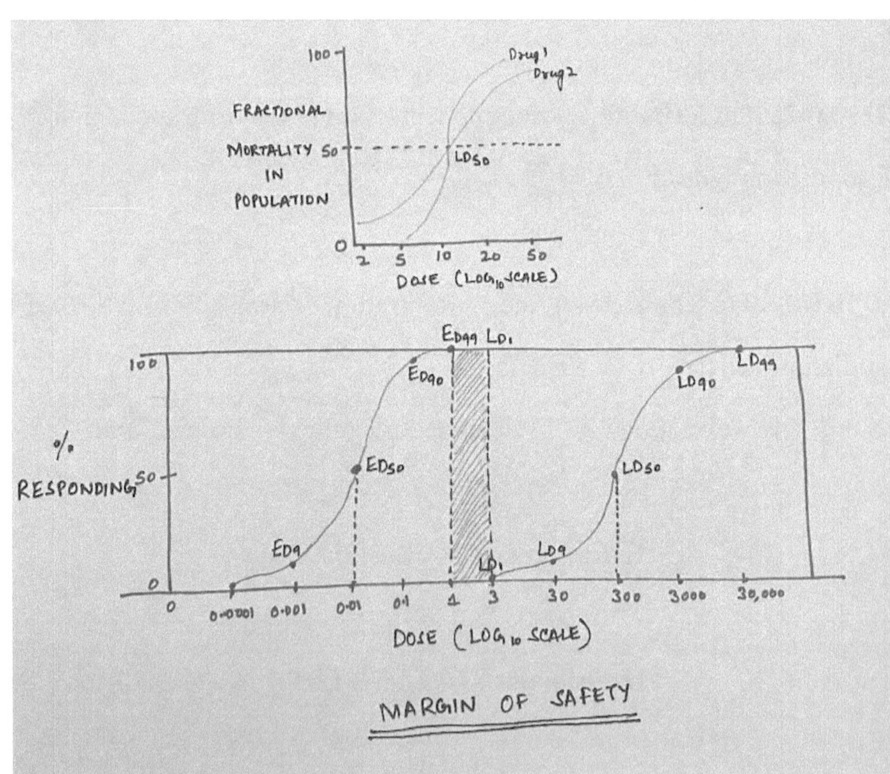

TOXICOKINETICS

- Excessive drug exposure is very harmful and easily adversely affects the Pharmacokinetics- ADME (Absorption, Distribution, Metabolism and Excretion) of a drug

- Factors affecting drug Absorption during toxic states are- Modified release drug dosage forms, delayed gastric emptying, pylorospasm, enterohepatic circulation and Pharmacobezoar (pharmaceutical medications conglomerate into a mass in the gut)

- Drug distribution during drug overdose encompasses parameters like plasma protein binding, pH influences and volume of distribution of drugs.

- Drug biotransformation in drug overdose is highly affected. First order kinetics switches to zero order kinetics with drug overdose. Saturated metabolic pathways shunt to alternative pathways and produce toxic metabolites. Active metabolites of drugs could turn to be more poisonous in nature.

- Drug transporters play a crucial role in elimination of "Xenobiotics" during this phase of toxicity.

Toxicity Classification

Side effects are undesirable effects away and far from normal therapeutic effects but still the drug may be continued for treatment.

Adverse drug effects occur at therapeutic drug dose

Toxic drug effects occur at supratherapeutic drug dose

- **On-target** - when drug reacts with its primary pharmacological target/receptor. It is dose dependent. E.g. Barbiturate binding to GABA mediated Chloride channels in overdose produce excessive sedation, coma and death.

- **Off-target**- when a drug reacts with a secondary pharmacological target/ receptor. It is generally seen during pre clinical studies and als in post marketing surveillance. E.g. Terfenadine in overdose blocks K+ channels in the heart leading to arrhythmias, apart from affecting normal H1 receptor

- **Biological activation**- when a drug is biologically activated to a toxic metabolite capable of deranging normal physiological systems. E.g. acetaminophen biologically activates to toxic NAPQI

- **Hypersensitivity Reactions**- it is an immune mediated response.

  - ☐ **Type 1 -Anaphylactic reactions**- these are mediated by IgE antibodies. Receptors on mast cells or basophils bind Fc portion of IgE, if Fab binds an antigen, mediators like histamines, PGs, LTs etc are released and lead to responses like edema, inflammation, vasodilation, etc. E.g. urticaria, food allergy, anaphylactic shock, etc.

- ☐ **Type 2- Cytolytic Reactions-** these are mediated by IgG and IgM. The complement system is activated. Cells in circulation are most affected. E.g. hemolytic anaemia caused by penicillin.

- ☐ **Type 3- Arthus Reaction-** these are mediated by IgG. Antigen antibody complexes are formed. Complement is fixed. Destructive inflammatory response known as "Serum Sickness" occurs with deposition of complexes in vasculature. The affected person shows a variety of signs and symptoms like skin eruptions, arthralgia, fever and lymph node involvement, etc. E.g. common antibiotics.

- ☐ **Type 4- Delayed Hypersensitivity Reactions-** these are mediated by sensitised T Lymphocytes and macrophages. Lymphokines are produced, and inflammatory reactions are generated. E.g. Contact dermatitis by poison Ivy

- **Idiosyncratic Reactions-** it is generally individual Specific and rare in occurrence. Though difficult to comprehend, these are immunotoxicological reactions with a background of strong pharmacogenetic basis. E.g. Steven Johnson syndrome, Toxic Epidermal Necrolysis.

Drug Interactions

Drug-drug interactions are a result of taking more than one medication simultaneously. These can be of two types:

- **Pharmacokinetic Interactions-** when ADME of one drug is modified by another.

   Absorption is affected (Ranitidine, an antacid may raise stomach pH and increase absorption of basic drugs like triazolam), there is involvement of drug transporters like P-gp, OAT and BCRP (inhibition of P-glycoprotein increases absorption and bioavailability), interactions occur at plasma protein binding site. Drugs highly bound to plasma proteins like warfarin, sulfonamides, valproic acid, etc can compete and displace less bound drugs from PPB sites. These drugs also exhibit toxicity in overdose. Metabolism is affected with involvement of hepatic CYPs. Inducers and Inhibitors can turn out to be game changers. Elimination is also affected. Lithium clearance is dependent on renal excretion.

- **Pharmacodynamic Interactions-** receptors are involved and they are of many types

Increased Effect **AGONISM**	Decreased Effect **ANTAGONISM**
ADDITION Combined effect is the sum of effect of each drug given separately	***PHYSIOLOGICAL*** Opposite effects produced by two drugs on the same physiological mechanics i.e. receptor is different
SYNERGISM Combined effects is more than the individual drug effect	***CHEMICAL*** Neutralisation of effects when two chemicals react together
POTENTIATION A no-effect drug can accentuate the response of another drug in its presence.	***RECEPTOR*** One drug blocks the other drug on the same receptor by competing or acting as an Allosteric site.

POISONING

- **Poisoning** may occur Intentionally (self harm, recreation, misuse, harm to others) or unintentionally (young children, exposure in the environment, occupation and Treatment mistakes and Iatrogenic errors). Most common and serious poisonings are reported with sedatives, hypnotics, opioids, alcohols, street drugs, acetaminophen, calcium channel blockers, beta blockers, hypoglycemic drugs, antidepressants and antihistamines.

- **Prevention** of poisoning is very essential. Primary prevention goal is to decrease exposure to the poison. This can be done by changing the product formulation, by reducing manufacturing and sale of poisons and by preventing access to poison. Secondary goal is to minimise the effect/damage due to exposure to poison. This can be achieved by making laymen aware of poison control services.

- **Management** of poisoning involves tri step clinical approach like Stabilisation, Evaluation and treatment. ABCs (Airway, Breathing and Circulation maintenance), Toxidromes (groups of physical signs and symptoms of a particular poisoning) serve for diagnosis and further treatment options of the poisoning. Serum toxicology labs serve for quick diagnosis.

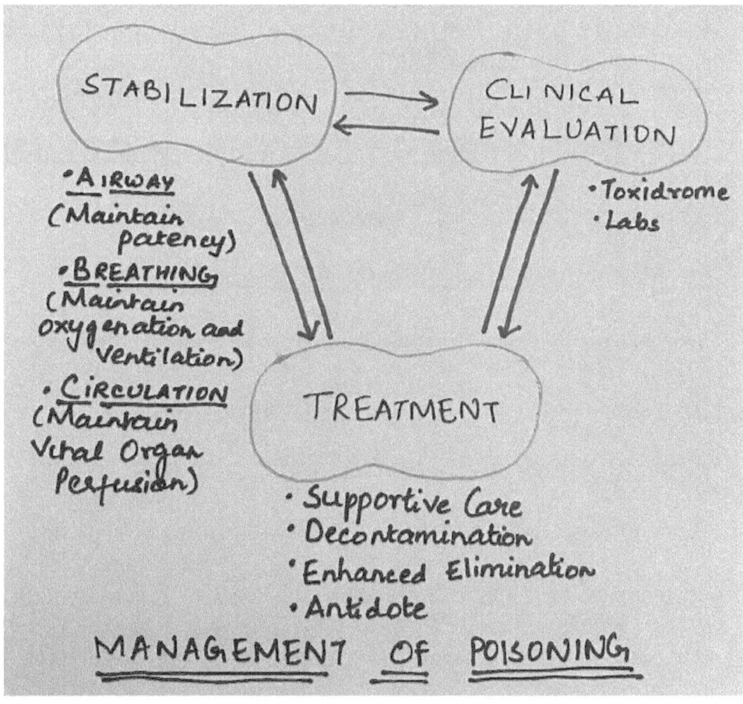

- **Treatment** involves supportive care like I.V. Fluids, antiemetics, benzodiazepines. Decontamination of the gut is done with the help of Activated Charcoal, whole bowel irrigation, Gastric emptying, Gastric lavage, Ipecac syrup and cathartics. Poison can be eliminated in a fast manner by Urinary pH modification and hemodialysis especially for serious cases like in toxicity of ethylene glycol, metformin, salicylate and valproic acid.

- **Antidotes** are very powerful chemical agents which can turn out to be life saviour in cases of life threatening poisonings. There are major three types of Antidotes like Chemical Antidotes (they bind to toxins and form inactive complexes which are excreted out of the body. E.g. Sugammadex given intravenously binds muscle relaxants like Rocuronium and aids in quick skeletal muscle recovery after surgery), Pharmacological Antidotes (toxin effect is antagonised at the receptor E.g. Naloxone is a competitive antagonist at mu-opioid receptors and is useful to reverse opioid toxicity) and Physiological/ Functional Antidotes (these use a different cellular mechanism to overcome poison effects. Antivenoms and chelating agents bind and form inactive complexes. Some antidotes alter metabolism E.g. Glucagon used for Beta blocker poisoning. Fomepizole use in ethylene glycol poisoning. Dispositional antidotes are capable of altering toxic metabolic pathways. E.g. Carnitine depletion in valproic acid poisoning.

- Some commonly used Antidotes
    1. N-Acetylcysteine (Acetaminophen)
    2. Calcium disodium EDTA (chronic lead poisoning)
    3. Dantrolene (malignant hyperthermia)
    4. Flumazenil (benzodiazepines)
    5. L-carnitine (valproic acid)
    6. Pyridoxine (hydrazine)
    7. Succimer (lead, mercury, arsenic)
    8. Leucovorin (methotrexate)

9. Fomepizole (ethylene glycol, methanol)

10. Naloxone (opioids)

11. Protamine (heparin)

12. Idarucizumab (dabigatran)

13. Pralidoxime-2 (organophosphate pesticides)

14. Hydroxocobalamin (cyanide)

15. Digoxin immune Fab (cardiac glycosides)

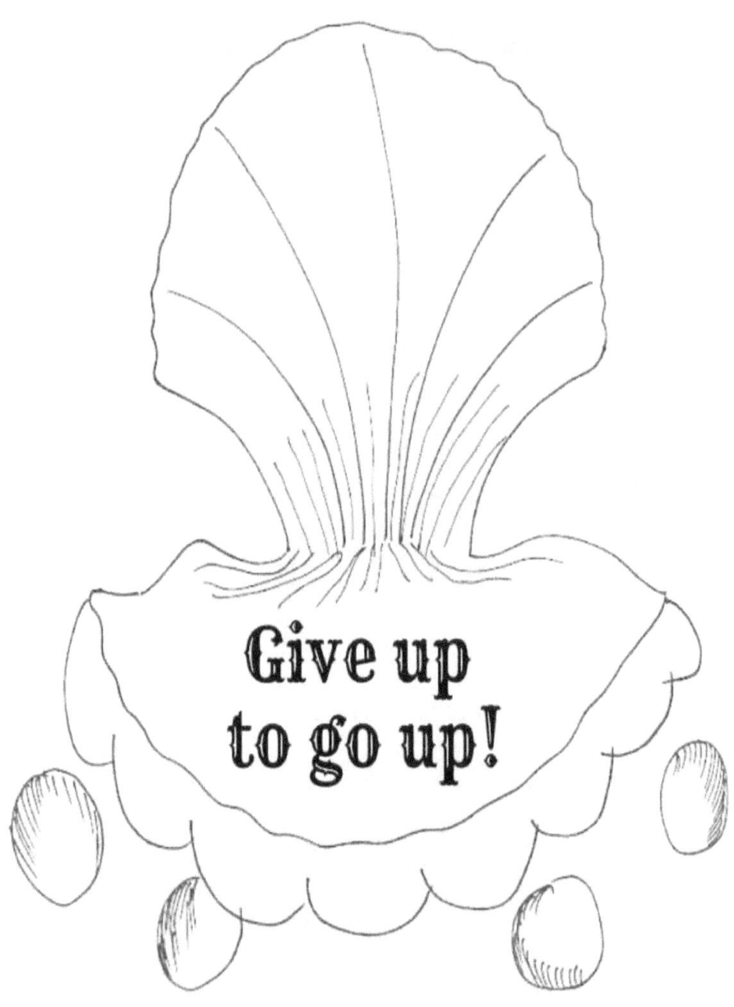
Give up
to go up!

References

1. *Goodman & Gilman's The Pharmacological Basis of therapeutics-14th Ed.*

2. *K.D. Tripathi's Essentials of Medical Pharmacology- 8th Ed.*

3. *Sharma & Sharma's Principles of Pharmacology-4th Ed.*

Abbreviations

1. AMA-American Medical Association & Council on Drugs

2. WHO-World Health Organisation

3. USA-United States of America

4. FDA- Food & Drug Administration

5. MDI-Metered Dose Inhaler

6. ACE-Angiotensin Converting Enzyme

7. HIV-Human Immunodeficiency Virus

8. HPMC- Hydroxypropyl methylcellulose

9. UK-United Kingdom

10. I.M.-Intra muscular

11. S.C.-Sub cutaneous

12. I.V.-Intra venous

13. TTS-Transdermal Therapeutic System

14. BCG-Bacille Calmette Guérin

15. ECF-Extracellular Fluid

16. SSRI-Selective Serotonin Reuptake Inhibitor

17. SERT- Serotonin Transporter

18. NET- Norepinephrine Transporter

19. SGLT-Sodium glucose co-transporter 2

20. PABA- Para aminobenzoic acid

21. GA- General Anaesthetics

22. EDTA- Ethylenediaminetetraacetic acid

23. DNA- De Oxy Ribo nucleic acid

24. ED50- Median Effective Dose

25. LD50-Median Lethal Dose

26. NSAID- Non Steroidal Anti Inflammatory Drugs

27. GABA- Gamma Amino Butyric Acid

28. IA- Intrinsic Activity

29. UDP- Uridine Diphosphate

30. GST- Glutathione-S Transferase

Afterword

Thanks for reading and making up this far!

Hope the book served your expectations and purpose!

And you can also subscribe on different social media like Twitter, Instagram, Facebook and Youtube.

And once again, don't forget to subscribe for my E-Newsletter on

www.ispharmacologydifficult.com

Acknowledgements

I especially want to mention a vote of thanks to my son who kept an eye all round the formatting, designing book cover and shaping of the book, positively critical yet highly supporting , though he never understood the ABC of the subject matter.

Next a great thanks to Mom and my brother for always being there by my side through thick and thin!

And never to forget , heartiest thanks to my lovely podcast audience, my auspicious listeners who brought me till here, of course, "You are the best!"

About The Author

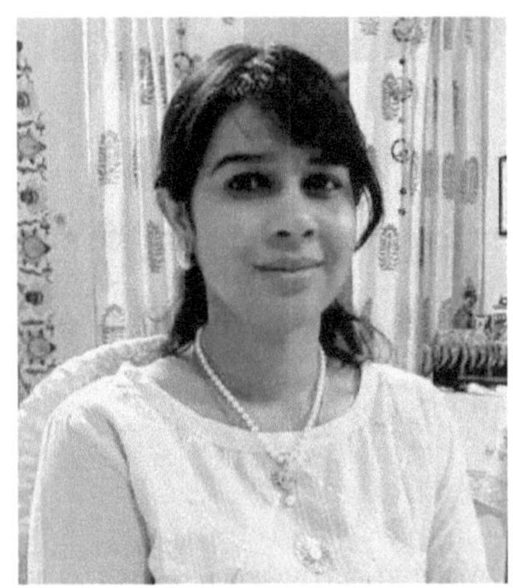

Radhika Vijay , MBBS, MD in Pharmacology belongs to Bikaner, Rajasthan, India. She is a faculty in Sardar Patel Medical College, Bikaner. She has always been an elite student since her school days. She has been teaching Medical Pharmacology for the last 10 years now and has touched different corners of this school -Teacher, Podcaster and Author now! Appreciator of everything brilliant and intelligent in life, she has tried to strive for the best in her educational endeavours. With an optimistic attitude and approach she believes in the value and power of time, prayers and purpose driven consistency as strong foundation elements in one's life!

You can connect:

Website: https://www.ispharmacologydifficult.com

Twitter : https://twitter.com/IsPharmacology

Facebook: https://www.facebook.com/ispharmacology.difficult.5

Instagram: https://www.instagram.com/ispharmacologydifficult/

Youtube:

https://www.youtube.com/channel/UC-LnUrZKlcBuQaLa2HDQOVg

9 798224 397839